The Changing Trends of Vector-Borne Diseases to Climate Change

Edited by

Jayalakshmi Krishnan
Vector Biology Research Laboratory
Department of Biotechnology
Central University of Tamil Nadu
Thiruvarur, India

Sigamani Panneer
Centre for the Study of Law and Governance
Jawaharlal Nehu University
New Delhi, India

P. Thiyagarajan
Department of Computer Science
Central University of Tamil Nadu
Thiruvarur, India

Balachandar Vellingiri
Department of Zoology
Central University of Punjab
Bathinda, India

&

Pradeep Kumar Srivastava
National Vector Borne Disease Control Programme
New Delhi, India

The Changing Trends of Vector Borne Diseases to Climate Change

Editors: Jayalakshmi Krishnan, Sigamani Panneer, P. Thiyagarajan, Balachandar Vellingiri and Pradeep Kumar Srivastava

ISBN (Online): 979-8-89881-276-8

ISBN (Print): 979-8-89881-277-5

ISBN (Paperback): 979-8-89881-278-2

Published by Bentham Science Publishers Pte. Ltd. Singapore, in collaboration with Eureka Conferences, USA. All Rights Reserved.

First published in 2025.

need for a court order if at any point you breach any terms of this License Agreement. In no event will any delay or failure by Bentham Science Publishers in enforcing your compliance with this License Agreement constitute a waiver of any of its rights.

3. You acknowledge that you have read this License Agreement, and agree to be bound by its terms and conditions. To the extent that any other terms and conditions presented on any website of Bentham Science Publishers conflict with, or are inconsistent with, the terms and conditions set out in this License Agreement, you acknowledge that the terms and conditions set out in this License Agreement shall prevail.

Bentham Science Publishers Pte. Ltd.
No. 9 Raffles Place
Office No. 26-01
Singapore 048619
Singapore
Email: subscriptions@benthamscience.net

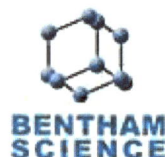

BENTHAM SCIENCE

CONTENTS

FOREWORD

Vector-borne illnesses have become a significant public health concern in recent years, highlighting the complex relationship between climate change and human health. The rising global temperatures, shifting rainfall patterns, and extreme weather events are influencing the geographical distribution and seasonality of many vectors, such as mosquitoes, ticks, and mites, which in turn affect the transmission dynamics of diseases they carry. As we stand on the brink of unprecedented environmental changes, it is vital to understand how climate change will reshape the landscape of infectious diseases.

This book, "The Changing Trends of Vector-Borne Diseases to Climate Change," provides a comprehensive exploration of how climate change is influencing some of the most significant vector-borne diseases affecting humans. By focusing on diseases such as dengue, malaria, scrub typhus, Kyasanur Forest Disease (KFD), and Crimean-Congo Hemorrhagic Fever (CCHF), the authors present a detailed examination of the environmental shifts that are expanding the range of these pathogens, altering their epidemiology, and posing new challenges for control and prevention.

Each chapter delves into a specific disease, examining the relationship between climate variability and its vector ecology, transmission patterns, and public health impact. By highlighting the urgent need for innovative strategies in disease surveillance, vector control, and public health infrastructure, this book aims to provide insights into how we can mitigate the growing threat of climate-induced vector-borne diseases.

As climate change continues to accelerate, the need for interdisciplinary research, global cooperation, and robust public health planning has never been more critical. I hope that the knowledge contained in this book will serve as a valuable resource for researchers and public health professionals alike as we face the challenges ahead.

With a greater understanding of the complex relationship between climate change and vector-borne diseases, we can work toward safeguarding human health in a rapidly changing world.

Rajesh Banu J.
Department of Biotechnology
Central University of Tamil Nadu
Thiruvarur, Tamil Nadu, India

PREFACE

Climate change has emerged as one of the most significant global challenges of our time, influencing ecosystems, public health, and human livelihoods. Among its many impacts, the shifting patterns of vector-borne diseases present a critical concern. As temperatures rise, precipitation patterns change, and extreme weather events become more frequent, the habitats and behaviors of vectors such as mosquitoes, ticks, and mites are undergoing significant transformations. These changes have profound implications for the spread of diseases like dengue, malaria, Crimean-Congo Hemorrhagic Fever (CCHF), Kyasanur Forest Disease (KFD), and scrub typhus.

This book explores the complex relationship between environmental changes and the epidemiology of vector-borne diseases. Each chapter examines a specific disease in the context of climate variability, providing insights into how fluctuations in temperature, humidity, and ecological dynamics are altering the geographical distribution and incidence of these illnesses. From the highlands where scrub typhus is making unexpected inroads to the emergence of KFD in regions previously unaffected, the book underscores the urgent need for a multidisciplinary approach to understanding the effects of climate change on public health.

Through detailed case studies, the book highlights how rising temperatures expand the range of vectors, creating new public health challenges and complicating efforts to control outbreaks. With a focus on diseases such as dengue, malaria, KFD, CCHF, and scrub typhus, this volume offers a comprehensive exploration of the complexities associated with vector-borne diseases in the era of climate change, providing invaluable insights for researchers, public health officials, and policymakers working to protect vulnerable populations.

Jayalakshmi Krishnan
Vector Biology Research Laboratory
Department of Biotechnology, Central University of Tamil Nadu
Thiruvarur, India

Sigamani Panneer
Centre for the Study of Law and Governance
Jawaharlal Nehu University
New Delhi, India

P. Thiyagarajan
Department of Computer Science
Central University of Tamil Nadu
Thiruvarur, India

Balachandar Vellingiri
Department of Zoology
Central University of Punjab
Bathinda, India

&

Pradeep Kumar Srivastava
National Vector Borne Disease Control Programme
New Delhi, India

List of Contributors

Jayalakshmi Krishnan Vector Biology Research Laboratory, Department of Biotechnology, Central University of Tamil Nadu, Thiruvarur, India

Joel Jaison Vector Biology Research Laboratory, Department of Biotechnology, Central University of Tamil Nadu, Thiruvarur, India

R Narendar Vector Biology Research Laboratory, Department of Biotechnology, Central University of Tamil Nadu, Thiruvarur, India

Rajalakshmi Anbalagan Vector Biology Research Laboratory, Department of Biotechnology, Central University of Tamil Nadu, Thiruvarur, India

S.K. Farhat Vector Biology Research Laboratory, Department of Biotechnology, Central University of Tamil Nadu, Thiruvarur, India

S Binduja Vector Biology Research Laboratory, Department of Biotechnology, Central University of Tamil Nadu, Thiruvarur, India

CHAPTER 1

Climate Change and Vector-Borne Diseases in General

Rajalakshmi Anbalagan[1] and **Jayalakshmi Krishnan**[1,*]

[1] *Vector Biology Research Laboratory, Department of Biotechnology, Central University of Tamil Nadu, Thiruvarur, India*

Abstract: Many arthropod species, including ticks, fleas, sand flies, mosquitoes, triatomine bugs, and black flies, serve as vectors for numerous diseases that affect humans and animals. These vectors transmit pathogens such as bacteria, viruses, and protozoa, which cause diseases like dengue fever, West Nile Virus, Lyme disease, and malaria. As cold-blooded animals, arthropod vectors are highly sensitive to fluctuations in climatic factors. Climate change significantly impacts several aspects of vector biology and ecology, including survival and reproduction, abundance and distribution, pathogen development and survival, as well as spatiotemporal distribution. Generally, climate change is a crucial factor influencing the survival, reproduction, distribution, and density of disease vectors, subsequently affecting the epidemiology of vector-borne diseases.

Keywords: Arthropods, Climate changes, Diseases, Distribution, Pathogens, Vector.

INTRODUCTION

Climate Change and Vector-Borne Diseases

Climate change is directly contributing to a range of humanitarian emergencies, including heatwaves, wildfires, floods, tropical storms, and hurricanes. These natural disasters are not only becoming more frequent but are also increasing in scale and intensity. The increasing severity of these events underscores the critical need for robust climate action and disaster preparedness strategies to mitigate their impact on vulnerable populations.

The change in climatic conditions, including an increase in heat waves, floods, and storms, has had a significant impact on human health. The evolving zoonotic

* **Corresponding author Jayalakshmi Krishnan:** Vector Biology Research Laboratory, Department of Biotechnology, Central University of Tamil Nadu, Thiruvarur, India; E-mail: jayalakshmi@cutn.ac.in

diseases and other vector-borne diseases have also played a major role in the changing effects of climate change [1].

The climatic factors that directly influence VBDs ecosystems are primarily temperature and rainfall. These factors play a crucial role in the life cycles of vectors and pathogens, as well as in the environments [2]. The transmission of VBDs requires a vector population, and diseases caused by pathogens such as parasites, viruses, bacteria, and in some cases, nematodes [3]. A vector is known to be an organism acting as a vehicle, which transmits or carries the pathogen from infected vector hosts to the uninfected hosts. Major global VBDs have been identified by the World Health Organization (WHO) and other research. Malaria, transmitted by *Anopheles* (*An.*) mosquitoes, remains one of the deadliest VBDs worldwide. Dengue, spread by *Aedes* mosquitoes, causes severe flu-like illness and sometimes leads to deadly complications. *Aedes* mosquitoes also transmit chikungunya, causing fever and severe joint pain. Yellow fever, a viral hemorrhagic disease, is spread by *Aedes* and *Haemagogus* mosquitoes. Zika spreads primarily by *Aedes* mosquitoes, and it can cause birth defects when transmitted from a pregnant woman to her fetus. Lymphatic filariasis is caused by parasitic worms transmitted through the bites of infected mosquitoes, leading to severe swelling and disability. Leishmaniasis, which is spread by sandflies, can cause skin sores or affect internal organs. Japanese encephalitis is a viral infection spread by mosquitoes carrying the Japanese encephalitis virus, which can cause inflammation of the human brain. These diseases pose significant public health challenges and contribute to substantial morbidity and mortality worldwide, as claimed by WHO.

Human activities, such as fossil burning, deforestation, and industrial processes, have led to an increase in greenhouse gases and caused an impact on ecosystems and biodiversity. Direct consequences of climate change, which are easier to observe, include excessive weather events such as hurricanes, floods, droughts, and changes in temperature and rainfall patterns. These events can have direct and visible impacts on human and ecological systems. Indirect consequences of climate change are also visible but can be equally overwhelming. One important indirect consequence is the alteration of the endemic range of parasitic diseases. Climate change can lead to shifts in the distribution of disease vectors (such as mosquitoes, ticks, and tsetse flies) and their reservoir hosts, as shown in Fig. (**1**) [4].

Non-climatic Factors

Several other factors have also been implicated in the emergence and recurrence of vector-borne diseases. The major non-climatic factors include urbanization, international trade, global human populations, travel-intensive livestock keeping systems, modernization of agricultural practices, and the proliferation of reservoirs. Studies on climate change and its impact on vector-borne diseases have also highlighted the effects of agricultural practices on human health. Several studies have reported that infectious diseases and human-induced land-use changes in agricultural practices are significantly linked. Agricultural works are associated with emerging zoonotic diseases, with more than 50% of human cases. Development projects, such as irrigation and the construction of dams, have also affected vector population densities, inducing the reappearance of zoonotic diseases (*e.g.*, Rift Valley Fever) [5 - 10].

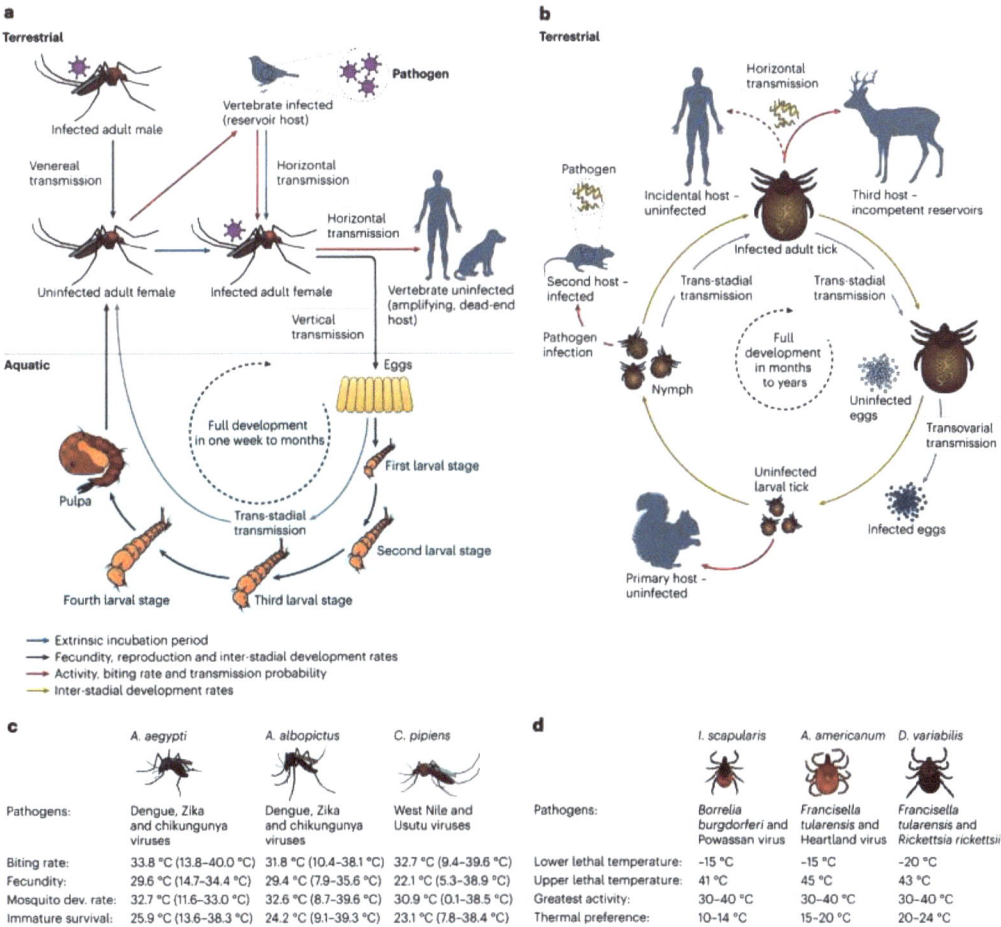

	A. aegypti	A. albopictus	C. pipiens			I. scapularis	A. americanum	D. variabilis
Pathogens:	Dengue, Zika and chikungunya viruses	Dengue, Zika and chikungunya viruses	West Nile and Usutu viruses	Pathogens:		Borrelia burgdorferi and Powassan virus	Francisella tularensis and Heartland virus	Francisella tularensis and Rickettsia rickettsii
Biting rate:	33.8 °C (13.8–40.0 °C)	31.8 °C (10.4–38.1 °C)	32.7 °C (9.4–39.6 °C)	Lower lethal temperature:		−15 °C	−15 °C	−20 °C
Fecundity:	29.6 °C (14.7–34.4 °C)	29.4 °C (7.9–35.6 °C)	22.1 °C (5.3–38.9 °C)	Upper lethal temperature:		41 °C	45 °C	43 °C
Mosquito dev. rate:	32.7 °C (11.6–33.0 °C)	32.6 °C (8.7–39.6 °C)	30.9 °C (0.1–38.5 °C)	Greatest activity:		30–40 °C	30–40 °C	30–40 °C
Immature survival:	25.9 °C (13.6–38.3 °C)	24.2 °C (9.1–39.3 °C)	23.1 °C (7.8–38.4 °C)	Thermal preference:		10–14 °C	15–20 °C	20–24 °C

Fig. (1). Impact of human activities and climate change on vector-borne diseases.
Source: [de Souza *et al.*, 2024]

MALARIA

Malaria is the most common parasitic disease worldwide, transmitted by the *Anopheles* mosquito. In 2022, there were approximately 249 million cases of malaria, with 608,000 malaria-related fatalities. The African Region accounted for 94% of malaria cases and 95% of malaria-related deaths during that year [1]. *Plasmodium (P.) falciparum* is indeed responsible for the mainstream of malarial cases, particularly the severe forms that can be life-threatening. On the other hand, *P. vivax* is also a significant cause of malaria, accounting for about 8% of estimated cases globally. *P. vivax* is more prevalent in regions outside of sub-Saharan Africa, such as Asia and Latin America, and is known for causing recurring infections due to its ability to form dormant liver stages called hypnozoites [11]. Climatic factors, particularly temperature, significantly influence the survival and longevity of mosquitoes and impact the rate at which parasites multiply within their vectors. In colder regions, mosquitoes and parasites have evolved strategies to survive winter conditions, while in warmer regions they adapt to endure dry seasons. The climate-related factors (temperature and moisture) play crucial roles in shaping the population dynamics of *Anopheles* mosquitoes, influencing their distribution, abundance, and capacity to transmit malaria.

Anopheles Mosquito

Anopheles is a genus of mosquitoes that transmits malaria diseases and is found worldwide, especially in tropical and subtropical regions. *Anopheles* mosquitoes are primary vectors of malaria. Female mosquitoes transmit *Plasmodium* parasites to humans through bites during their blood feeding.

Lifecycle

Egg: Laid in water and hatch into larvae within 2-3 days.

Larva: Aquatic stage that feeds on microorganisms; lasts about 7-14 days.

Pupa: Non-feeding, transitional stage lasting 2-3 days.

Adult: Emerges from the pupa, ready to feed and reproduce.

Only female *Anopheles* mosquitoes bite humans, as they require blood for egg development, while male mosquitoes feed on nectar. *Anopheles* desire clean water bodies, such as ponds, rice fields, cement tanks, and syntax tanks. Adult Anopheles mosquitoes are attracted to dark, sheltered areas for resting during the day [12].

MALARIA ERADICATION

The simple phrase 'malaria eradication' obscures the inherent complexity posed by six distinct *Plasmodium* species. While the pathogenesis of *P. falciparum* is well-defined, *P. vivax* presents a rapidly growing challenge. Furthermore, comprehensive technical data remain scarce for *P. malariae*, *P. ovale* subspecies, and *P. knowlesi*. Consequently, it is widely acknowledged that current tools are insufficient for malaria elimination [13].

CLIMATE CHANGE - MALARIA

Temperature also affects the duration of each life stage (egg, larva, pupa, adult) of the mosquito. Higher temperatures typically accelerate development, while lower temperatures slow it down. The development of malaria parasites (*Plasmodium spp.*) within the mosquito is also temperature-dependent. For example, *P. falciparum* requires a specific temperature range to develop fully within the mosquito vector [14, 15].

Climate change induced by human activities is indeed expected to increase the burden of vector-borne diseases, particularly malaria. Climate-based models predict that rising temperatures and changing rainfall patterns will extend the malaria season in many sub-Saharan African regions [16].

DENGUE

Dengue is a mosquito-borne viral infection prevalent in warm, tropical climates. The infection is caused by any one of four closely related viruses, known as serotypes (DENV-1, DENV-2, DENV-3, and DENV-4) [17]. *Aedes* mosquitoes, particularly *Ae.*, primarily transmit dengue. [*Ae.*] *aegypti* and *Ae. Albopictus* are common in tropical and subtropical regions, including Southeast Asian countries, the Pacific Islands, the Caribbean, Africa, and parts of South America [18]. The incidence of dengue is positively associated with ecological factors such as temperature, relative humidity, and rainfall in various regions around the world, including the Americas [3].

Dengue and Climate Change

Climate change is a critical factor influencing the transmission dynamics of dengue [19]. Higher temperatures can accelerate the life cycle of mosquitoes, reducing the time needed for them to mature from larvae to adults. This can lead to larger mosquito populations. Additionally, higher temperatures can accelerate the replication of the dengue virus within the mosquito, thereby reducing the incubation period and increasing the likelihood of transmission [20, 21]. Rainfall can create more breeding sites for mosquitoes, as many mosquito species, including *Ae. aegypti* (the primary vector for dengue) and *Ae. albopictus* lay their eggs in stagnant water [22]. However, continuous rainfall washes down the larvae and temporarily decreases the mosquito population. On the contrary, drought conditions can force people to store water, creating ideal breeding sites for mosquitoes [23]. There is evidence of an epidemic of dengue cases, with a rise in climatic conditions such as temperature, rainfall, and relative humidity [24].

CHIKUNGUNYA

Aedes mosquito carrying Chikungunya Virus (CHIKV) of the family alphavirus (family *Togaviridae*) is a worldwide public health threat. Chikungunya fever is usually characterized by severe polyarthralgia and myalgia, often leading to chronic infections, such as rheumatic diseases [25]. The first origination of CHIKV was reported in Africa over 500 years ago, with Asia reporting cases later. With circulating strains of CHIKV, major outbreaks have occurred across the globe with no vaccines available. Both rural and urban areas have reported current or previous CHIKV transmissions and outbreaks.

Chikungunya and Climate Change

Based on certain modeling studies, climate change has increased the incidence of *Aedes*-borne diseases [27]. Various research studies have been developed in the field of vector ecology and its control to figure out and monitor the changing trends and patterns of VBDs, which is very important and crucial for addressing the challenges arising from climate change factors and the transmission of diseases such as chikungunya and Dengue [28].

YELLOW FEVER

Yellow fever is a viral-borne infectious disease transmitted to humans by the bite of infected. *Ae. aegypti* mosquitoes. The virus originates from specific regions in South America and Africa. In 1648, the first outbreak of Yellow fever was reported on the Yucatan Peninsula. The diseases are spread by a biting mosquito that breeds around houses (domestic) and in forests/jungles, or both habitats. Yellow fever is a highly threatening disease, with a global health burden. Frequently, yellow fever is exported by infected travelers to many countries. However, under specific climate conditions, yellow fever can easily spread given the presence of necessary mosquito species and an animal reservoir to maintain the virus [1]. After 3-4 days of infection, people start showing symptoms, including headache, backache, muscle ache, fever, and chills. After 3-6 days of the infection, around 12% of people go on to develop serious illness such as jaundice, bleeding, shock, organ failure, and in some cases, lead to death [12].

Climate Change in Yellow Fever

Approximately 10% of climate and weather-related factors influence zoonotic diseases. Higher temperatures can enhance the replication rate of the yellow fever virus within mosquitoes, making them more efficient vectors. This can increase the likelihood of transmission to humans [30].

ZIKA

Zika is a mosquito-borne flavivirus disease. *Ae. Aegypti* act as a primary vector mosquito, transmitting diseases. Zika Virus (ZIKV) is also transmitted by sexual intercourse, during pregnancy, and from a mother to fetus [31, 32]. ZIKV is closely related to other flaviviruses, like Dengue virus, West Nile Virus, Yellow Fever Virus, and Japanese Encephalitis virus. In 1947, the first isolation was performed in Uganda, and ZIKV was first isolated from a sentinel rhesus monkey. In 2016, approximately 440,000 to 1,300,000 cases were reported across parts of Brazil during the outbreak [33, 34]. World Health Organization (WHO) announced Zika Virus as "a public health emergency of global angst." On February 1st, 2016, drastic actions to decrease the infection in pregnant women and women of reproductive age were exposed [35].

Climate Change in Zika

The relationship between climate change and ZIKV adds an extra layer of complexity. Certainly, the 2016 Zika outbreak prompted research into the climatic factors influencing the transmission of Zika virus compared to dengue [33]. Some of the major combining experimental and modeling approaches to minimize temperature for ZIKV transmission by *Ae. aegypti* is approximately 5°C, which is higher than that of dengue virus [36]. Research on systematic assessment of upcoming temperatures is a promising tool for determining the appropriate transmission and distribution of ZIKV and its risk to human health [27].

Aedes Mosquito

Aedes mosquitoes are primarily found in urban areas and near human populations. The dengue mosquito lays its eggs in wet containers, such as discarded plastic waste, a syntax tank, a cement tank, a discarded tyre, and a coconut shell. Inside the home, they lay eggs in refrigerator trays, flower pots, *etc*. The eggs hatch when they are in flow with water, and the eggs can remain stable for three months under optimal conditions. The adult mosquitoes rest indoors in dark areas. The increased safety of these indoor resting spots enhances their life expectancy, which in turn raises the likelihood of them surviving long enough to acquire and transmit viruses from one human to another. This behavior plays an important role in the transmission of diseases, such as dengue [37].

Aedes aegypti

Ae. (*Stegomyia*) *Aegypti Linnaeus* 1762 is a widely distributed mosquito species and the primary vector of dengue, chikungunya, Zika, and yellow fever in humans. They spread throughout the tropical and subtropical areas in the world. It is highly anthropophilic in nature, preferring only human blood meals and also bread in human habitats.

Aedes albopictus

Ae. albopictus (Skuse) are medically important vectors found in 129 countries worldwide. Climate change predictions indicate that the *Ae. albopictus*, is likely to continue its successful spread beyond its current geographical boundaries. Mainly, rainfall patterns can create more suitable breeding sites. Increased rainfall can lead to more standing water, while some areas may become more susceptible due to changes in humidity levels. Additionally, increased global travel and trade can facilitate the spread of *Ae. albopictus* eggs and larvae, often transported through goods like used tires and ornamental plants. Therefore, monitoring and controlling the spread of *Ae. albopictus* is crucial in the context of climate change [38].

LYMPHATIC FILARIASIS

Lymphatic Filariasis (LF), also known as elephantiasis, is spread by infected mosquitoes and is a neglected tropical disease caused by *Brugia malayi*, *Brugia timori*, and *Wuchereria bancrofti*. The parasites are transmitted by various species of mosquitoes, which vary geographically. Overall, 120 million people are affected by LF. It is endemic in 72 countries worldwide, with continued endemicity observed in several nations within the Americas, including Brazil, Guyana, Haiti, and the Dominican Republic [1]. According to the World Health Organization (WHO) classifies LF is classified as the second cause for long-term disability, followed by mental illness. The Global Programme to Eliminate LF (GPELF) was founded in 2000 with the goal of global elimination of LF. Though the goal was not fully realized, important strides have been made in reducing LF endemicity worldwide. GPELF strategies consist of Mass Drug Administration (MDA) [39]. Numerous attempts were made to encourage defensive immune responses against LF introducing the parasite into an ectopic site, infecting with a strain that remains subclinical in the host, vectors and parasites with the live worms attenuated through artificial techniques such as X-irradiation or γ-irradiation, chemically abbreviated infections, or injecting the metabolites derived from the culture supernatants of live worms, yield unreliable results [40, 41].

Climate Change- Lymphatic Filariasis

The development and survival of mosquito vectors are influenced by temperature, and higher temperatures can accelerate their life cycle, leading to increased mosquito populations. Thus, enhance the transmission of the filarial parasites. The development rate of the filarial parasites within the mosquito vectors is temperature-dependent. Warmer temperatures can reduce the development time of parasites, increasing the likelihood of transmission [41].

JAPANESE ENCEPHALITIS

Japanese Encephalitis Virus (JEV) is transmitted through *Culex* mosquitoes, especially to pigs and wading birds. More than 40 JE cases were identified in the Australian mainland and south in 2021 and the mid-2022 period [42 - 44]. JEV infections were absent during the winter season and were again identified on the Australian mainland in November 2022, hence strongly suggesting that the virus is permanently present [45].

Culex Mosquito

The genus *Culex* is quite diverse, with 768 species categorized into 26 subgenera. These mosquitoes are important vectors for several diseases, including West Nile virus, Japanese encephalitis, and filariasis. The diversity within the genus allows them to inhabit a wide range of environments, contributing to their role in disease transmission.

The life cycle of *Culex* mosquitoes, like other mosquitoes, involves numerous stages:

Eggs: Adult female *Culex* mosquitoes lay eggs on fresh or stagnant water. Eggs are often laid in clusters, forming a raft that can contain several hundred eggs.

Larvae: The eggs hatch into larvae, commonly known as "wrigglers," which live in water. They come to the surface to breathe and feed on organic matter and microorganisms.

Pupae: After several molts, the larvae develop into pupae, or "tumblers." The pupal stage is a transitional phase where the mosquito undergoes metamorphosis.

Adult Mosquitoes: Pupae eventually develop into adult, flying mosquitoes. Adult female mosquitoes search for blood meals from humans and animals. Blood is necessary for the production of eggs. After feeding, they lay eggs. This life cycle is distinctive for many mosquito species and is crucial for understanding their role in disease transmission and for developing effective control measures [12].

Climate Changes in Japanese Encephalitis

Climate change has led to the global development of JE, driven by increases in travel, rice cultivation, pig farming, and agricultural practices. Climate change is assumed to be a key driver of the emergence of JEV in all temperate regions. Primarily, the heavy rainfall suitable for wetland conditions leads to higher mosquito populations, highlighting the interplay between the spread of vector-borne diseases and different climates [46].

SCRUB TYPHUS

Scrub typhus is a zoonotic, vector-borne disease transmitted by the bite of infected chigger mites that carry the bacterium *Orientia tsutsugamushi*. The disease is widespread in regions of Australia, Southeast Asian countries, the Pacific Islands, and occasionally in the Middle East. Key environments for scrub typhus transmission contain areas with scrub vegetation, such as forest clearings, riverbanks, grassy fields, deserts, and rainforests. In the U.S., scrub typhus is rare and naturally seen in travellers who have visited endemic regions. Scrub typhus, with its clinical symptoms, includes fever, headache, body aches, and sometimes a rash like a lesion. If not treated, the disease can become rigorous and even fatal, but it is treatable with antibiotics like doxycycline.

Severe Complications

The high fatality rate in scrub typhus cases, particularly among hospitalized patients, is associated with complications such as:

Pulmonary Complications

- Acute Respiratory Distress Syndrome (ARDS)
- Pneumonia
- Pulmonary edema

Cardiac Complications

- Myocarditis
- Pericarditis
- Heart failure

Hepatic Complications

• Hepatitis
• Jaundice

Neurological Complications

• Meningoencephalitis
• Confusion
• Seizures

Renal Complications

• Acute kidney injury
• Renal failure

Prognosis and Management

Early diagnosis and prompt treatment with antibiotics such as doxycycline or azithromycin are crucial for preventing these severe outcomes. Delay in treatment is often associated with a higher risk of developing these complications and an increased mortality rate.

Precautionary measures

Preventing scrub typhus involves reducing exposure to areas where the chigger mites are present. Diseases can be prevented by using insect repellent containing DEET, wearing long-sleeved shirts and long pants, avoiding walking through tall grass and brush, applying permethrin to clothing and gear, and ensuring good environmental hygiene to minimize rodent habitats near living areas. Early diagnosis and treatment are crucial for managing scrub typhus successfully [18].

Climate change in Scrub typhus

The prevalence of scrub typhus, an arthropod-borne disease caused by *O. tsutsugamushi*, is highly climate-dependent. The various meteorological factors,

such as temperature, relative humidity, and rainfall, increase the incidence of scrub typhus.

Limited Research on Nonlinear and Lag Effects in Scrub Typhus

• Few studies have investigated the nonlinear and lag effects of meteorological factors on scrub typhus on a monthly timescale [51].
• Only one study has explored these effects on a weekly timescale, although the

specific meteorological thresholds that increase scrub typhus risk were not clearly defined [52].

In Tamil Nadu, the older people, farmers, agricultural workers, and females (homemakers) were at higher risk for scrub typhus.

1. **Relative Humidity (RH)**: Increase in relative humidity was associated with a 7.6% increase in monthly scrub typhus cases, with a 95% Confidence Interval (CI) ranging from 5.4% to 9.9%. This suggests that higher humidity levels may create favorable conditions for the vectors or the disease itself, leading to more cases.
2. **Rainfall**: A 1 mm increase in rainfall is associated with a 0.5% to 0.7% rise in monthly ST clinical cases. This indicates that rainfall can influence the incidence of scrub typhus, potentially by affecting vector breeding sites or other environmental conditions that are conducive to the disease's spread.

These insights emphasize the importance of considering environmental factors, such as humidity and rainfall, in understanding and predicting the dynamics of scrub typhus transmission [53].

Control strategy of vector-borne diseases

1. Environmental Management

- **Source Reduction**: Eliminate breeding sites of vectors, such as stagnant water bodies for mosquitoes. This includes clearing drainage systems, removing standing water, and disposing of waste properly.
- **Urban Planning**: Design cities to minimize vector habitats, such as ensuring good drainage, adequate water supply, and sanitary housing.

2. Biological Control

- **Predators and Pathogens**: Use biological agents like fish [*e.g., Gambusia*], bacteria [*e.g., Bacillus thuringiensis israelensis*], or fungi to reduce vector populations.
- **Sterile Insect Technique (SIT)**: Release sterilized male mosquitoes that do not produce offspring, thereby reducing the number of future generations.

3. Chemical Control

- **Insecticides**: Utilize chemical insecticides (*e.g.*, pyrethroids, DDT) in public health interventions, such as Indoor Residual Spraying (IRS) and space spraying, during outbreaks.
- **Larvicides**: Apply chemicals to water sources to kill mosquito larvae, reducing

adult populations.
- **Insecticide-Treated Nets (ITNs):** Bed nets treated with insecticides which protect and reduce disease transmission, especially for malaria.

4. Personal Protection

- **Repellents**: Use of topical insect repellents, wearing protective clothing, and installing window screens to reduce bites.
- **Insecticide-Treated Clothing**: Wearing clothes impregnated with long-lasting insecticides.

5. Vaccination and Medication

- **Vaccines**: Develop and administer vaccines against diseases like yellow fever, dengue (Dengvaxia), and Japanese encephalitis.
- **Prophylaxis**: Use preventive medication, such as antimalarials for travelers and those in endemic regions.

6. Surveillance and Early Detection

- **Vector Monitoring**: Regular surveillance of vector populations to track density and species distribution.
- **Disease Surveillance**: Early diagnosis and reporting of vector-borne diseases to prevent outbreaks.
- **Climate Data Use**: Leverage climate data to predict and respond to outbreaks driven by weather changes.

7. Community Involvement

- **Public Awareness Campaigns**: Educate communities on reducing vector habitats and using protective measures.
- **Community Clean-up Drives**: Engage communities in sanitation and source reduction efforts.

8. Genetic Control

- **Gene Editing**: Utilize gene-editing technologies, such as CRISPR, to reduce vector populations or render vectors incapable of transmitting diseases.

9. Integrated Vector Management (IVM)

- **Combination Approach**: Employ a combination of the above strategies tailored to local epidemiological conditions. IVM aims to use the most effective, sustainable, and environmentally friendly approaches available [54].

Future Impact of Climate Change on Vector Borne Diseases

For the upcoming period, the impact of climate change on vector-borne diseases is predictable to be important, as changes in temperature, precipitation, and humidity directly change the division and activities of vectors [such as mosquitoes, fleas, and ticks] that transmit diseases like malaria, dengue, Zika, Lyme disease, and others.

1. Expanded Geographic Range

- **Warming temperatures:** Extend the habitats of many vectors, which allows them to survive in areas that were formerly too cold. This means diseases like malaria and dengue, traditionally confined to tropical regions, could spread to more temperate regions, including parts of Europe and North America.
- For example, Malaria transmitted by *Anopheles* mosquitoes, as well as Dengue, Zika, and Chikungunya transmitted by *Aedes*, may start to thrive in higher altitudes and latitudes.

2. Changes in Disease Transmission Seasons

- Warmer temperatures may lead to longer transmission seasons for many vector-borne diseases. In areas where malaria transmission was previously seasonal, longer warm periods could extend the duration during which mosquitoes are active and able to transmit the disease.
- **Dengue and Chikungunya** thrive in hot, humid climates, posing a year-round threat in many regions, as conditions favor longer breeding cycles for these mosquitoes.

3. Increased Vector Abundance

- Changes in the rainfall patterns can create more breeding sites for mosquitoes. The increased rainfall leads to more stagnant water, which is ideal for mosquito breeding. At the same time, drought conditions can concentrate water sources and increase the density of mosquito populations around remaining water bodies.
- Warmer temperatures also increase the lifespan of mosquitoes, potentially leading to higher populations and accelerating the incubation of viruses within the vectors.

4. Higher Disease Transmission Efficiency

- Warmer temperatures can also speed up the development of pathogens within vectors. *Plasmodium* parasites, which cause malaria, develop more rapidly inside mosquitoes at higher temperatures, potentially increasing the rate at which mosquitoes become infectious. Thus leads to higher transmission rates in regions.

5. Emergence of New Disease Hotspots

• Regions that have not historically experienced vector-borne diseases, such as parts of Europe, North America, and East Asia, may see the emergence of new disease hotspots due to changing climates. For example, Lyme disease may spread further north into Canada and Russia as ticks expand their range.

6. Urbanization and Human Impact

• Rapid urbanization, combined with climate change, may exacerbate disease transmission. Urban areas with poor infrastructure and inadequate drainage may become breeding grounds for mosquitoes due to increased rainfall and poor water management.
• Population displacement due to extreme weather events, such as floods and droughts, could also lead to the spread of diseases as people move to new areas where they may not have immunity to local diseases.

7. Potential for Increased Outbreaks

• Increased weather variability, including extreme events such as hurricanes, floods, and heatwaves, may disrupt ecosystems and public health systems, leading to an increase in outbreaks of diseases like dengue, malaria, and Zika in both endemic and newly affected regions.

8. Impacts on Control and Mitigation Efforts

• Climate change may demoralize effective vector control efforts. For example, the use of insecticide-treated nets and indoor residual spraying may be less valuable as mosquitoes adapt to new environmental conditions.

• Public health systems may face greater strain as they have to manage increasing disease burdens in both traditional and newly affected areas [55].

Limitations

There were various considerable limitations. First, predictive modeling of diseases based solely on climate change is inherently defective. The use of control measures, such as mass drug administration, safe drinking water, and sanitation, serves as a key strategy to reduce the global burden of NTDs. Climate change, including changes in temperature and rainfall, is a commonly identified factor in various records. The various trends depicted in this review would suggest that climate change may contribute to a shift and drift in disease transmission and distribution of several vectors and NTDs, reflecting the changing trends of latitudinal and longitudinal shifts. However, while this chapter aims to identify these geographical areas and populations at risk of incursion or re-emergence and discuss the impact on specific vulnerable populations and/or territories, the identified gaps and limitations meant that this was not well achieved by the changing patterns of climate change.

Mathematical Modelling of Climate Change and VBDs

The distribution of VBDs is imperfect, with climatic conditions favouring warmer regions of the globe, and global warming also threatens to alter the geographic area for malaria transmission and other VBDs. A wide variety of process-based models, based on mathematical models, have been proposed, particularly those driven by highly nonlinear weather conditions. More commonly, both global and local environmental changes drove the initial emergence of *P. falciparum* as a major human pathogen in tropical Africa thousands of years ago, and the disease has a long and complex history throughout [57]. The climatic variables in the modelling are a critical issue to be considered. The maximum, minimum, mean temperature, rainfall, and relative humidity indices have been included in mathematical modeling [58].

CONCLUSION

In this chapter, we have explained climate change in vector-borne diseases, disease transmission in vectors and hosts, vector capacity, and vector control. Climate change is significantly reshaping the backdrop of VBDs, posing substantial public health challenges. The warming temperatures, altered rainfall patterns, and increased incidence of tremendous weather events are increasing the habitats of vectors such as mosquitoes and ticks. This extension enables these vectors to proliferate in earlier non-endemic regions, thereby increasing the incidence and geographical range of diseases such as malaria, dengue, Zika, and Lyme disease. Our exploration has shed light on climate change, vectorial capacity, and disease transmission. Urbanization and deforestation complicate the disruption of ecosystems and enable the movement of pathogens from one place to another. In conclusion, the impact of climate change on VBDs necessitates a comprehensive approach, including effective control strategies to address this growing threat through enhanced projection modeling and early warning systems to anticipate outbreaks. Public health campaigns must focus on increasing awareness, developing preventive strategies, and strengthening health infrastructure in exposed communities.

REFERENCES

[1]   Dengue and severe dengue. 2024. Available from: https://www.who.int/health-topics/dengue-a-d-severe-dengue

[2]   Fouque F, Reeder JC. Impact of past and on-going changes on climate and weather on vector-borne diseases transmission: a look at the evidence. Infect Dis Poverty 2019; 8(1): 51.
[http://dx.doi.org/10.1186/s40249-019-0565-1] [PMID: 31196187]

[3]   Semenza JC, Rocklöv J, Ebi KL. Climate change and cascading risks from infectious disease. Infect Dis Ther 2022; 11(4): 1371-90.
[http://dx.doi.org/10.1007/s40121-022-00647-3] [PMID: 35585385]

[4]   Short EE, Caminade C, Thomas BN. Climate change contribution to the emergence or re-emergence of parasitic diseases. Infect Dis (Auckl) 2017; 10: 1178633617732296.
[http://dx.doi.org/10.1177/1178633617732296] [PMID: 29317829]

[5]   McFarlane R, Sleigh A, McMichael A. Land-use change and emerging infectious disease on an island continent. Int J Environ Res Public Health 2013; 10(7): 2699-719.
[http://dx.doi.org/10.3390/ijerph10072699] [PMID: 23812027]

[6]   Gottdenker NL, Streicker DG, Faust CL, Carroll CR. Anthropogenic land use change and infectious diseases: a review of the evidence. EcoHealth 2014; 11(4): 619-32.
[http://dx.doi.org/10.1007/s10393-014-0941-z] [PMID: 24854248]

[7]   Kock RA. Vertebrate reservoirs and secondary epidemiological cycles of vector-borne diseases. Rev Sci Tech 2015; 34(1): 151-63.
[http://dx.doi.org/10.20506/rst.34.1.2351] [PMID: 26470455]

[8]   Shah HA, Huxley P, Elmes J, Murray KA. Agricultural land-uses consistently exacerbate infectious disease risks in Southeast Asia. Nat Commun 2019; 10(1): 4299.
[http://dx.doi.org/10.1038/s41467-019-12333-z] [PMID: 31541099]

[9]   Rohr JR, Barrett CB, Civitello DJ, *et al.* Emerging human infectious diseases and the links to global food production. Nat Sustain 2019; 2(6): 445-56.
[http://dx.doi.org/10.1038/s41893-019-0293-3] [PMID: 32219187]

[10]   Pepin M, Bouloy M, Bird BH, Kemp A, Paweska J. Rift Valley fever virus (*Bunyaviridae: Phlebovirus*): an update on pathogenesis, molecular epidemiology, vectors, diagnostics and prevention. Vet Res 2010; 41(6): 61.
[http://dx.doi.org/10.1051/vetres/2010033] [PMID: 21188836]

[11]   Baird JK. Neglect of *Plasmodium vivax* malaria. Trends Parasitol 2007; 23(11): 533-9.
[http://dx.doi.org/10.1016/j.pt.2007.08.011] [PMID: 17933585]

[12]   CDC. Mosquitoes. Life Cycle of *Anopheles* Mosquitoes. 2024. Available from: https://www.cdc.gov/mosquitoes/about/life-cycle-of-anopheles-mosquitoes.html

[13]   Tanner M, Greenwood B, Whitty CJM, *et al.* Malaria eradication and elimination: views on how to translate a vision into reality. BMC Med 2015; 13(1): 167.
[http://dx.doi.org/10.1186/s12916-015-0384-6] [PMID: 26208740]

[14]   Depinay JMO, Mbogo CM, Killeen G, *et al.* A simulation model of African Anopheles ecology and population dynamics for the analysis of malaria transmission. Malar J 2004; 3(1): 29.
[http://dx.doi.org/10.1186/1475-2875-3-29] [PMID: 15285781]

[15]   Rossati A, Bargiacchi O, Kroumova V, Zaramella M, Caputo A, Garavelli PL. Climate, environment and transmission of malaria. Infez Med 2016; 24(2): 93-104.
[PMID: 27367318]

[16]   Tanser FC, Sharp B, le Sueur D. Potential effect of climate change on malaria transmission in Africa. Lancet 2003; 362(9398): 1792-8.
[http://dx.doi.org/10.1016/S0140-6736(03)14898-2] [PMID: 14654317]

[17]   Wong JM, Adams LE, Durbin AP, *et al.* Dengue: A growing problem with new interventions. Pediatrics 2022; 149(6): e2021055522.
[http://dx.doi.org/10.1542/peds.2021-055522] [PMID: 35543085]

[18]   CDC. Dengue. How Dengue Spreads. 2024. Available from: https://www.cdc.gov/dengue/transmission/index.html

[19]   Ramasamy R, Surendran SN. Global climate change and its potential impact on disease transmission by salinity-tolerant mosquito vectors in coastal zones. Front Physiol 2012; 3: 198. Available from: https://www.frontiersin.org/journals/physiology/articles/10.3389/fphys.2012.00198/full
[http://dx.doi.org/10.3389/fphys.2012.00198] [PMID: 22723781]

[20]   Chen SC, Hsieh MH. Modeling the transmission dynamics of dengue fever: Implications of temperature effects. Sci Total Environ 2012; 431: 385-91.
[http://dx.doi.org/10.1016/j.scitotenv.2012.05.012] [PMID: 22705874]

[21]   Earnest A, Tan SB, Wilder-Smith A. Meteorological factors and El Niño Southern Oscillation are independently associated with dengue infections. Epidemiol Infect 2012; 140(7): 1244-51.
[http://dx.doi.org/10.1017/S095026881100183X] [PMID: 21906411]

[22]   Hales S, de Wet N, Maindonald J, Woodward A. Potential effect of population and climate changes on global distribution of dengue fever: an empirical model. Lancet 2002; 360(9336): 830-4.
[http://dx.doi.org/10.1016/S0140-6736(02)09964-6] [PMID: 12243917]

[23]   Johansson MA, Cummings DAT, Glass GE. Multiyear climate variability and dengue--El Niño southern oscillation, weather, and dengue incidence in Puerto Rico, Mexico, and Thailand: a longitudinal data analysis. PLoS Med 2009; 6(11): e1000168.
[http://dx.doi.org/10.1371/journal.pmed.1000168] [PMID: 19918363]

[24]   Patz JA, Martens WJ, Focks DA, Jetten TH. Dengue fever epidemic potential as projected by general circulation models of global climate change. Environ Health Perspect 1998; 106(3): 147-53.
[http://dx.doi.org/10.1289/ehp.98106147] [PMID: 9452414]

[25]   Kramer IM, Pfeiffer M, Steffens O, *et al.* The ecophysiological plasticity of *Aedes aegypti* and *Aedes albopictus* concerning overwintering in cooler ecoregions is driven by local climate and acclimation capacity. Sci Total Environ 2021; 778: 146128.
[http://dx.doi.org/10.1016/j.scitotenv.2021.146128] [PMID: 34030376]

[26]   Wahi N. Land acquisition in India: A review of supreme court cases from 1950 to 2016. Rochester, NY: Social Science Research Network 2017. Internet Available from: https://papers.ssrn.com/abstract=3915345

[27]   Ryan SJ, Carlson CJ, Mordecai EA, Johnson LR. Global expansion and redistribution of *Aedes*-borne virus transmission risk with climate change. PLoS Negl Trop Dis 2019; 13(3): e0007213.
[http://dx.doi.org/10.1371/journal.pntd.0007213] [PMID: 30921321]

[28]   George AM, Kargbou A, Wadsworth R, Kangbai JB. Trends and seasonal variations for confirmed

[29]   Ogden NH, Radojevic′ M, Wu X, Duvvuri VR, Leighton PA, Wu J. Estimated effects of projected climate change on the basic reproductive number of the Lyme disease vector *Ixodes scapularis*. Environ Health Perspect 2014; 122(6): 631-8.
[http://dx.doi.org/10.1289/ehp.1307799] [PMID: 24627295]

[30]   Brady OJ, Johansson MA, Guerra CA, *et al.* Modelling adult *Aedes aegypti* and *Aedes albopictus* survival at different temperatures in laboratory and field settings. Parasit Vectors 2013; 6(1): 351.
[http://dx.doi.org/10.1186/1756-3305-6-351] [PMID: 24330720]

[31]   Abrams RPM, Solis J, Nath A. Therapeutic approaches for zika virus infection of the nervous system. Neurotherapeutics 2017; 14(4): 1027-48.
[http://dx.doi.org/10.1007/s13311-017-0575-2] [PMID: 28952036]

[32]   Basu R, Tumban E. Zika Virus on a Spreading Spree: what we now know that was unknown in the

1950's. Virol J 2016; 13(1): 165.
[http://dx.doi.org/10.1186/s12985-016-0623-2] [PMID: 27716242]

[33] Carlson CJ, Dougherty ER, Getz W. An ecological assessment of the pandemic threat of zika virus. PLoS Negl Trop Dis 2016; 10(8): e0004968.
[http://dx.doi.org/10.1371/journal.pntd.0004968] [PMID: 27564232]

[34] Gyawali N, Bradbury RS, Taylor-Robinson AW. The global spread of Zika virus: is public and media concern justified in regions currently unaffected? Infect Dis Poverty 2016; 5(1): 37.
[http://dx.doi.org/10.1186/s40249-016-0132-y] [PMID: 27093860]

[35] Oladapo OT, Souza JP, De Mucio B, de León RGP, Perea W, Gülmezoglu AM. WHO interim guidance on pregnancy management in the context of Zika virus infection. Lancet Glob Health 2016; 4(8): e510-1.
[http://dx.doi.org/10.1016/S2214-109X(16)30098-5] [PMID: 27211476]

[36] Tesla B, Demakovsky LR, Mordecai EA, Ryan SJ, Bonds MH, Ngonghala CN, *et al.* Temperature drives Zika virus transmission: evidence from empirical and mathematical models. Proc Biol Sci 2018.
[http://dx.doi.org/DOI: 10.1098/rspb.2018.0795] [PMID: 30111605]

[37] *Aedes aegypti* - Factsheet for experts. 2017. Available from: https://www.ecdc.europa.eu/en/disease-vectors/facts/mosquito-factsheets/aedes-aegypti

[38] Ahebwa A, Hii J, Neoh KB, Chareonviriyaphap T. *Aedes aegypti* and *Aedes albopictus* (Diptera: Culicidae) ecology, biology, behaviour, and implications on arbovirus transmission in Thailand: Review. One Health 2023; 16: 100555.
[http://dx.doi.org/10.1016/j.onehlt.2023.100555] [PMID: 37363263]

[39] Cromwell EA, Schmidt CA, Kwong KT, *et al.* The global distribution of lymphatic filariasis, 2000–18: a geospatial analysis. Lancet Glob Health 2020; 8(9): e1186-94.
[http://dx.doi.org/10.1016/S2214-109X(20)30286-2] [PMID: 32827480]

[40] Babayan SA, Allen JE, Taylor DW. Future prospects and challenges of vaccines against filariasis. Parasite Immunol 2012; 34(5): 243-53.
[http://dx.doi.org/10.1111/j.1365-3024.2011.01350.x] [PMID: 22150082]

[41] Kwarteng A, Ahuno ST. Immunity in filarial infections: Lessons from animal models and human studies. Scand J Immunol 2017; 85(4): 251-7.
[http://dx.doi.org/10.1111/sji.12533] [PMID: 28168837]

[42] Heffelfinger JD, Li X, Batmunkh N, *et al.* Japanese encephalitis surveillance and immunization — asia and western pacific regions, 2016. MMWR Morb Mortal Wkly Rep 2017; 66(22): 579-83.
[http://dx.doi.org/10.15585/mmwr.mm6622a3] [PMID: 28594790]

[43] Buescher EL, Scherer WF, Rosenberg MZ, Gresser I, Hardy JL, Bullock HR. Ecologic studies of Japanese encephalitis virus in Japan. II. Mosquito infection. Am J Trop Med Hyg 1959; 8(6): 651-64.
[http://dx.doi.org/10.4269/ajtmh.1959.8.651] [PMID: 13805722]

[44] Gould DJ, Edelman R, Grossman RA, Nisalak A, Sullivan MF. Study of Japanese encephalitis virus in Chiangmai Valley, Thailand. IV. Vector studies. Am J Epidemiol 1974; 100(1): 49-56.
[http://dx.doi.org/10.1093/oxfordjournals.aje.a112008] [PMID: 4842558]

[45] Care AGD of H and A. Japanese encephalitis. Australian Government Department of Health and Aged Care. 2023 Available from: https://www.health.gov.au/diseases/japanese-encephalitis

[46] Pendrey CGA, Martin GE. Japanese encephalitis clinical update: Changing diseases under a changing climate. Aust J Gen Pract 2023; 52(5): 275-80.
[http://dx.doi.org/10.31128/AJGP-07-22-6484] [PMID: 37149766]

[47] Leishmaniasis immunopathology—impact on design and use of vaccines, diagnostics and drugs | Seminars in Immunopathology. 2024. Available from: https://link.springer.com/article/10.1007/s00281-020-00788-y

[48]   Rogers ME. The role of leishmania proteophosphoglycans in sand fly transmission and infection of the Mammalian host. Front Microbiol 2012; 3: 223.
[http://dx.doi.org/10.3389/fmicb.2012.00223] [PMID: 22754550]

[49]   Van Bocxlaer K, Caridha D, Black C, *et al.* Novel benzoxaborole, nitroimidazole and aminopyrazoles with activity against experimental cutaneous leishmaniasis. Int J Parasitol Drugs Drug Resist 2019; 11: 129-38.
[http://dx.doi.org/10.1016/j.ijpddr.2019.02.002] [PMID: 30922847]

[50]   Sáez VD, Morillas-Márquez F, Merino-Espinosa G, *et al.* Phlebotomus langeroni Nitzulescu (Diptera, Psychodidae) a new vector for Leishmania infantum in Europe. Parasitol Res 2018; 117(4): 1105-13.
[http://dx.doi.org/10.1007/s00436-018-5788-8] [PMID: 29404748]

[51]   Li W, Niu Y, Ren H, Sun W, Ma W, Liu X, *et al.* Climate-driven scrub typhus incidence dynamics in South China: A time-series study. 2022. Available from: https://dissem.in/p/131844770/climate-driven-scrub-typhus-incidence-dynamics-in-south-china-a-time-series-study/

[52]   Lu J, Liu Y, Ma X, Li M, Yang Z. Impact of meteorological factors and southern oscillation index on scrub typhus incidence in guangzhou, Southern China, 2006–2018. Front Med (Lausanne) 2021; 8: 667549.
[http://dx.doi.org/10.3389/fmed.2021.667549] [PMID: 34395468]

[53]   D'Cruz S, Perumalla SK, Yuvaraj J, Prakash JAJ. Geography and prevalence of rickettsial infections in Northern Tamil Nadu, India: a cross-sectional study. Sci Rep 2022; 12(1): 20798.
[http://dx.doi.org/10.1038/s41598-022-21191-7] [PMID: 36460687]

[54]   Adelman ZN, Tu Z. Control of mosquito-borne infectious diseases: Sex and gene drive. Trends Parasitol 2016; 32(3): 219-29.
[http://dx.doi.org/10.1016/j.pt.2015.12.003] [PMID: 26897660]

[55]   Caminade C, McIntyre KM, Jones AE. Impact of recent and future climate change on vector-borne diseases. Ann N Y Acad Sci 2019; 1436(1): 157-73.
[http://dx.doi.org/10.1111/nyas.13950] [PMID: 30120891]

[56]   de Souza WM, Weaver SC. Effects of climate change and human activities on vector-borne diseases. Nat Rev Microbiol 2024; 22(8): 476-91.
[http://dx.doi.org/10.1038/s41579-024-01026-0] [PMID: 38486116]

[57]   Eikenberry SE, Gumel AB. Mathematical modeling of climate change and malaria transmission dynamics: a historical review. J Math Biol 2018; 77(4): 857-933.
[http://dx.doi.org/10.1007/s00285-018-1229-7] [PMID: 29691632]

[58]   Naish S, Dale P, Mackenzie JS, McBride J, Mengersen K, Tong S. Climate change and dengue: a critical and systematic review of quantitative modelling approaches. BMC Infect Dis 2014; 14(1): 167.
[http://dx.doi.org/10.1186/1471-2334-14-167] [PMID: 24669859]

CHAPTER 2

Climate Change and Scrub Typhus

S.K. Farhat[1] and **Jayalakshmi Krishnan[1,*]**

[1] Vector Biology Research Laboratory, Department of Biotechnology, Central University of Tamil Nadu, Thiruvarur, India

Abstract: Vector-borne diseases are infections transmitted to humans through the bite of vectors, which are transmitted by arthropods such as mosquitoes, ticks, fleas, and mites. These zoonoses have become a major public health alarm affecting millions of people globally. According to recent reports from the World Health Organization (WHO), the estimated number of cases of vector-borne diseases, namely malaria and Dengue, was 247 million and 390 million, respectively, with cases reported globally. The change in environmental conditions like climate change with variations in the temperature, humidity, rainfall, and precipitation has impacted the change in disease dynamics. This chapter explores the relationship between the impact of climate change and Scrub typhus as well as the risk factors that contribute to Scrub typhus and climate change.

Keywords: Chigger mites, Climate change, Rickettsial infection, Scrub typhus, Seasonal change.

INTRODUCTION

According to the United Nations Framework Convention on Climate Change (UNFCCC), the term "climate change" is defined as the alterations in global temperature conditions that alter human activities and cause harm to the environment [1]. The use of industrialization and urbanization has led to the greenhouse effect, where the emission of harmful gases, such as CO_2, methane, and CFCs, thins the ozone layer by capturing these gases, thus leading to Global warming [2, 3]. Climate change leads to a rise in temperature and a change in rainfall patterns, affecting chigger mite vectors.

For any vector-borne zoonotic disease to occur, it requires an interaction of the epidemiological triad comprising the Agent, Host, and environment [4]. It is the basic model used in all epidemiological studies to identify the root cause of

---

* **Corresponding author Jayalakshmi Krishnan:** Vector Biology Research Laboratory, Department of Biotechnology, Central University of Tamil Nadu, Thiruvarur, India; E-mail: jayalakshmi@cutn.ac.in

Jayalakshmi Krishnan, Sigamani Panneer, P. Thiyagarajan, Balachandar Vellingiri & Pradeep Kumar Srivastava (Eds.)

disease transmission and facilitate its early detection and diagnosis. Upon disturbance in this triad, the so-called diseases known as epidemics, endemics, and pandemics cause havoc to the public health population.

Agent

The agent is the primary cause of the disease, primarily comprising infectious microorganisms such as bacteria, viruses, and parasites that cause illness. Eliminating or eradicating the agent will help control the disease at the primary level. The gram-negative bacterium *Orientia tsutsugamushi* is the agent of Scrub typhus, which is transmitted through the saliva of infected chigger mites [5].

Host

The host is the susceptible or vulnerable living animal or human on which these agents enter to complete their life cycle, thereby transmitting the pathogenic agents into human cells. Humans are the primary hosts of Scrub typhus, while some small mammals serve as secondary hosts [6]. Rodents, on the other hand, are the usual reservoirs that carry the larval chigger mites and are termed reservoir hosts, acting as natural reservoirs for *Orientia tsutsugamushi*, the bacterium responsible for the disease [7, 8]. Additionally, humans serve as incidental hosts when they come into contact with the chigger mites (larval stage of mites) that transmit the bacterium (Fig. **1**).

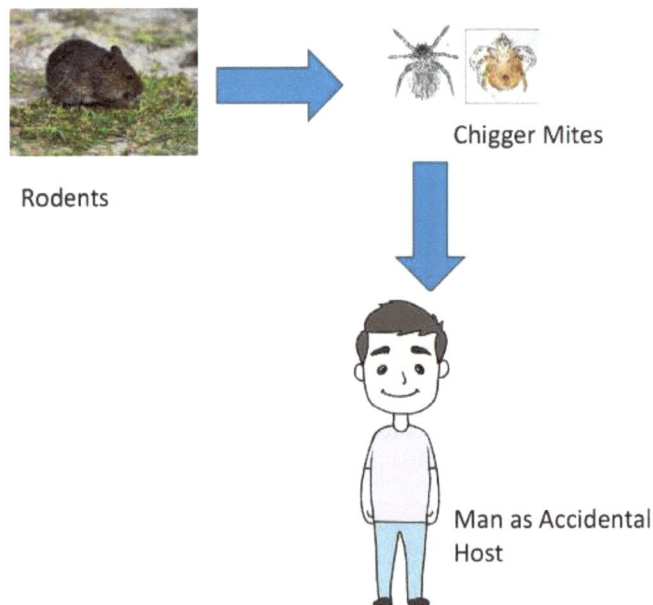

Chigger Mites

Rodents

Man as Accidental Host

Fig. (1). Lifecycle of scrub typhus.

Rodents (Primary Hosts/Reservoirs)

• *Rattus* **species** (rats)
• *Apodemus* **species** (field mice)
• *Bandicota* **species** (bandicoot rats)

These rodents are found in a wide range of habitats, from forests to farmlands and urban areas, and are the primary source of infection for the larval mites (chiggers) [9].

Chigger Mites (Vector)

Although not a "host," chigger mites (larval stage of **trombiculid mites**) play a crucial role as the vector of scrub typhus. The larvae feed on the blood of infected rodents and subsequently transmit the bacteria to humans. Notable species of chigger mites include [10, 11]:

• *Leptotrombidium deliense*
• *Leptotrombidium akamushi*

The mites remain infected for life, but they primarily feed on rodents. Humans are only incidental hosts when they come into contact with mite-infested environments, such as forests, scrublands, or farmlands.

Humans (Incidental Hosts)

Humans are not natural hosts for *Orientia tsutsugamushi*, but they become **incidental hosts** when exposed to infected chigger mites. This exposure often occurs in rural or forested areas, especially where human activities, such as farming, bring them into proximity with rodent populations or mite-infested environments [12].

Unlike rodents, humans do not contribute to the natural life cycle of the bacterium because they are not involved in its long-term transmission. However, scrub typhus can cause severe illness in humans, leading to fever, rash, and multi-organ complications if left untreated.

Other Mammals (Incidental Hosts)

While rodents are the primary hosts, other small mammals, such as shrews or wild animals, may also act as secondary or incidental hosts in some ecosystems [12 - 14]. However, they play a lesser role in the overall transmission dynamics compared to rodents and humans.

Role of Hosts in Scrub Typhus Transmission

- **Rodents** serve as natural reservoirs of the bacterium and play a crucial role in maintaining the transmission cycle.
- **Chigger mites** acquire the bacteria by feeding on infected rodents and then transmit the bacteria to other hosts (including humans).
- **Humans** are incidental hosts, infected only when they come into contact with mite-infested areas.

Environment

The external climatic conditions, such as temperature, humidity, and rainfall, influence the agent and the host in disease transmission. Scrub typhus is a seasonal disease that typically occurs during the monsoon and post-monsoon seasons. The grasslands, scrublands, and forests are the areas where dense bushes are present, thus enhancing the suitable conditions for the mite and creating mite islands [15].

In contrast to the environment, changes in external conditions affect the occurrence of vector-borne diseases. The triad will affect the cyclodevelopmental, cyclopropagative, and propagative life cycles of vectors, thus facilitating the rapid spread of disease transmission.

THE DISEASE - SCRUB TYPHUS

Scrub typhus is a rickettsial infection transmitted to humans through the bite of infected larval chiggers, which carry the gram-negative bacterium *Orientia tsutsugamushi* in their salivary glands. The disease, which was previously thought to be affecting the tsutsugamushi triangle, is now re-emerging and has notably become endemic throughout the Asian Pacific region [16], affecting all age groups, with approximately one billion people globally. The disease is primarily underdiagnosed or underreported due to its common clinical symptoms of fever, headache, myalgia, and vomiting, thus classifying the disease under Fever of Unknown Origin. The mortality rate of Scrub typhus is reported to be as high as around 30-35% when not treated and diagnosed timely.

A unique clinical sign, the presence of an Eschar, has made Scrub typhus recognizable from other vector-borne rickettsial infections [17, 18]. Another common clinical parameter observed in Scrub typhus infections is the deteriorating levels of thrombocytopenia (decreased platelet count), which can counteract Dengue cases, making it difficult to diagnose the disease [19]. The vector mite carrying the disease agent is taxonomically classified into the following [20]:

Classification:

Kingdom: Animalia

Phylum: Arthropoda

Subphylum: Chelicerata

Class: Arachnida

Subclass: Acari

Order: Acariformes

Suborder: Actinedida

Family: Trombiculidae

The Life Cycle

The life cycle of chigger mites comprises eggs, Larvae, Nymphs, and Adults. The female adult mites, after mating, lay eggs in the soil, which hatch into larvae within one to three weeks. The areas typically found for laying eggs are dense and bushy vegetation with high humidity and moisture areas where the environment is pleasant for the adults to lay eggs. Scrub typhus typically prefers warm and humid environmental conditions, found in both temperate and tropical regions. Female adults lay eggs in conditions, preferably with wet soil and dense vegetative regions [21].

Larva

After the hatching of the eggs, the larvae emerge from the egg, which is the only parasitic stage of the chigger mite's life cycle. The larvae are too tiny to be seen through the naked eye since they are very tiny (usually less than 0.3 mm) and are visible only under the microscope [22]. The larvae are differentiated from adults by their legs, as larvae have six legs, whereas adults have eight legs. Once the larvae hatch from the egg in the soil, they climb into the vegetation and attack their host (such as a human, bird, or small mammal). Although humans are the accidental hosts, rodents serve as reservoirs. They typically feed for about three to four days.

In rodents, the larval mites are found attached to the ear pinna and leg regions. In humans, they are found in hidden areas, such as the groin, near the finger folds, and genital areas, making them invisible to the naked eye. The larvae on the host's skin inject digestive enzymes, thus breaking down the host skin cells by causing itching and skin irritation in the host [23].

The hatching of the larvae depends on external environmental conditions, such as temperature, rainfall, and humidity. During the low temperatures, the larvae hatch faster than usual.

Nymph

The Nymph is the third part of the life cycle, where the larvae detach from the host and fall into the soil, thus molting into nymphs. Nymphs have eight legs and resemble adult mites, but are smaller and sexually immature. The nymph goes through several stages called protonymph, deutonymph, and tritonymph.

Adult

The adult chigger mites are eight-legged (four pairs) and free-living in the soil, measuring approximately 1-2 mm in length. Adult males and females lay eggs in the soil, thus completing the life cycle of the mites [21].

CLIMATE CHANGE AND SCRUB TYPHUS

The disturbance or change in environmental factors caused by the self-centered nature of anthropogenic activities has resulted in abrupt changes in the atmospheric environment, leading to the evolution of vector-borne diseases, which are noted to be a major public health concern [3]. Although the life cycle of vectors follows the cycle of egg-larvae-pupae/nymphs and adults, their development and habitats are entirely dependent on factors such as temperature, rainfall, humidity, and ecosystems in which they dwell. The change in these environmental factors will alter their ability to reproduce and thus hinder their role as vectors in transmitting the pathogens from the reservoir to the host. It is estimated that approximately 6.3 million people are living with the risk of vector-borne disease transmission, with more than 300 million cases and a death rate of around 700,000 annually [15, 24]. Seasonal fluctuations in climatic conditions play a pivotal role in vector-borne disease transmission and dynamics.

Rickettsial diseases are infections caused by bacteria of the genus Rickettsia, which are transmitted to humans through arthropods (mites, ticks, and fleas). Scrub typhus is one such Rickettsial infection transmitted to humans through the bite of infected larval chigger mites, which carry the gram-negative bacterium Orientia tsutsugamushi in their salivary glands, serving as vectors. The disease is endemic throughout the tsutsugamushi triangle, comprising parts of China, Japan, and Southeast Asian regions, including Thailand, Cambodia, Vietnam, Laos, and parts of Indonesia and Malaysia, with sero-prevalence ranging from 9.3% to 27.9% [25]. Although the disease shows a mortality of 1.4%- 6%, perhaps the timely differential diagnosis of Scrub typhus with its similar clinical manifestations has to be considered effectively [26].

Meteorology and Scrub Typhus

For studying the vector-borne disease transmission and bionomics of any rickettsial infections, such as Scrub typhus, public health professionals must delve into the meteorology, which involves studying the weather and atmospheric conditions of the current time and place. The influence of wind, rainfall, humidity, precipitation, and temperature together helps the development of both vectors and pathogens.

The endemicity of Scrub typhus, which ranges from temperate to tropical regions throughout the year, depends mainly on meteorological factors, including temperature, rainfall, precipitation, and relative humidity. It is noted that for every 1°C increase in monthly average temperature, humidity, and rainfall in China, there was a rise in Scrub typhus cases of 15.4%, 0.7%, and 12.6%, respectively [27]. The incidence of Scrub typhus cases varies according to the seasonal variations in regions ranging from temperate to tropical. The chigger mites that are engulfed by the eggs will search for their host, which can be rodents or humans, to feed on the nymphs and adults, which freely live in the soil. The cases of Scrub typhus usually peak during post-monsoon climates, especially in October and November, when bushes grow, creating shaded and humid locations that favor a suitable environment for chigger mites [15].

Rainfall and Scrub Typhus

Rainfall plays a significant role in the transmission of vector-borne diseases, such as scrub typhus, which is directly dependent on rodent populations and mite density [28]. It increases the availability of food sources for rodents and their living environment by growing bushes and shrubs, which serve as the primary hosts for the mites. An increase in rodent populations during and after monsoon seasons can lead to higher chigger populations.

An accelerated fall of rain on the plains eventually favors the suitable environment for vector-borne diseases such as Dengue, Malaria, Japanese Encephalitis (JE), Chikungunya caused by Arthropod mosquitoes, and other Rickettsial infections, namely, Kyasanur Forest Disease (KFD), Scrub typhus, and Murine Typhus caused by ticks, mites, and fleas. The use of entomological indices, such as the House Index, Bruteo Index, Container Index, and Pupal Index, during frequent dengue outbreaks has helped in containing the disease severity and making early predictions. The chigger mite index and flea index are the parameters to be measured to contain the disease outbreak [29].

Entomological indices

Assessing the entomological indices to control vectors and disease transmission is crucial during and before the occurrence of any vector-borne outbreaks. The indices vary according to the arthropods causing the disease, including ticks, mites, fleas, and mosquitoes.

The rickettsial infection, Scrub typhus, is measured through the Chigger index and Chigger infestation rate [22].

Chigger Index

• **Higher chigger index:** Indicates a higher density of chigger mites on hosts, increasing the likelihood of transmission to humans.
• **Lower chigger index**: Suggests fewer mites on host animals, which may correlate with a reduced risk of disease transmission.

Chigger Infestation Rate

• **High infestation rate**: Indicates that a large proportion of the rodent population is infested with chiggers, increasing the potential for scrub typhus transmission.
• **Low infestation rate**: Indicates fewer rodents are infested, suggesting a lower overall risk of transmission in the area.

The Seasonal Patterns

Due to the huge geographical diversity of India, the Scrub typhus endemic regions experience a diverse range of climates, with four main seasons affecting the disease pattern accordingly (Fig. **2**) [30, 31].

Winter (December-February)

The characteristic feature of this season is usually cold and dry, with the southern parts experiencing mild winters and the northern regions experiencing severe cold, often below the freezing point. The humidity is low, providing little comfort to humans and contributing to winter-borne occupational and other diseases.

Monsoon

Summer

Winter

Post-Monsoon

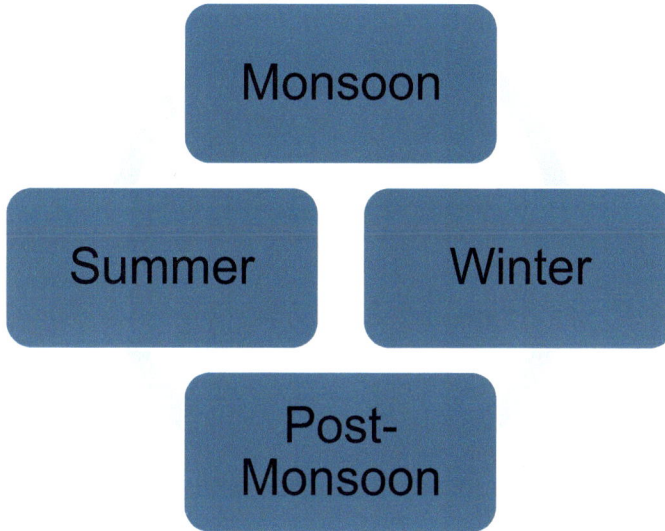

Fig. (2). Seasonal cycle of Scrub typhus cases.

Summer (March - June)

The characteristic feature of this season is usually hot and dry. These seasons experience extremely high temperatures exceeding 45°C (113°F). The coastal regions face high humidity. The season favors the vector habitat for their pleomorphic development and the completion of their life cycle.

Monsoon (June - September)

The characteristic feature of this season begins with high humidity, with temperatures ranging from 25°C to 35°C (77°F to 95°F), and usually heavy rainfall, leading to an increase in Scrub typhus incidence. The increased

vegetation and suitable environmental conditions during this period promote chigger activity, enhancing the chances of human contact with infected chiggers.

The southwest monsoon brings substantial rainfall to most parts of the country, with a spike in vector-borne disease cases.

Post-monsoon or Autumn (October - November)

The characteristic feature of this season typically begins with retreating monsoons and a decrease in rainfall. The temperature usually ranges from 20°C to 30°C (68°F to 86°F). Although some light showers occur, making the environment pleasant, they also favor the growth of environmental microorganisms. Even after the rains have stopped, the residual moisture in the environment can maintain favorable conditions for chiggers, sustaining the risk of transmission for several weeks or months.

Regional Variations

- **Northern Mountains:** Experience severe winters with heavy snowfall; summers are mild and pleasant, but scrub typhus cases emerge in the northern Himalayan regions.
- **Coastal Regions:** Moderate climate with less temperature variation, high humidity, and significant rainfall during the monsoon. During environmental disasters like floods, coastal regions are severely affected by vector-borne diseases.
- **Central India:** Hot and dry summers, moderate rainfall during the monsoon, and cool winters. These areas are vulnerable to all forms of diseases throughout the climatic conditions.
- **Desert Regions:** Extreme hot summers, cool winters, and scanty rainfall.

Henceforth, Scrub typhus is endemic throughout the Southeast Asian regions, affecting all the hooks and corners of the continent, irrespective of climate change [32].

Effect of Rainfall on Chiggers and Scrub Typhus

Habitat

Since the name Scrub typhus suggests the vernacular name Bush typhus, the Chigger mites that transmit the gram-negative bacterium Orientia tsutsugamushi to humans are found in dense populations in mite islands, where abundant bushes and grasses grow, especially during monsoons and post-monsoon rainfalls, making it a favorable habitat for rodents and spreading this endemic disease. The rodent burrows are the primary target for mite collection, as these rodents carry mites that occasionally shed chigger mites into the soil, where humans become accidental hosts [33].

Increased Humidity

Rainfall plays a role in increasing humidity levels, which in turn favors the Chigger mite population by enabling its life cycle to proceed faster. A Retrospective study conducted in Vellore showed a positive correlation between the mean relative humidity and the number of Scrub typhus cases, with a percentage increase of 55 to 89% [34]. The more humid the air is, the more discomfort it creates for humans, and conversely, it creates a comfort zone for vectors, which easily transport pathogens from the reservoir to the host, thereby completing their life cycle.

In general, the life cycle of the Trombiculid mites, from egg to adult, is supposed to be completed within 2-12 months, which varies according to changes in climatic conditions and patterns. The life cycle varies from temperate to tropical regions, with a shorter life cycle in tropical regions over the years [35].

Population Dynamics

Scrub typhus, once thought to be a rural disease, is now being spread to the urban population due to rapid urbanization, leading to the man-vector interaction [36]. Although both rural and urban settings have predominant habitats for chigger mite infestations, cases of Scrub typhus are at their peak. The change in environmental factors, such as rainfall, influences the population of rodents, which eventually increases the number of cases.

High Altitudes

People usually harbor infections like Scrub typhus when living at higher altitudes above 2500m above sea level. The adventurous trekkers visiting mountain ranges, as well as the sub-Himalayan and Himalayan people dwelling in the forest range for fossil fuels and daily activities, make them vulnerable to Scrub infections and other dermatological infections [37]. The literature has also noted hypoxia in Scrub typhus-infected patients, resulting in multi-organ dysfunction. The healthcare delivery system in India's hilly regions, with limited health resources, may result in cases being underreported and underdiagnosed.

RODENT DENSITY AND CLIMATE CHANGE

Vector-borne diseases, such as Lyme disease (Borrelioses), Malaria, Leptospirosis, and Rickettsial infections, are transmitted by arthropods, including mosquitoes, fleas, ticks, and mites, which feed on rodents for their survival by sucking the host's blood and completing their gonotrophic cycle, comprising blood feeding, egg laying, and egg development. The rapid growth of dense rodent populations will ultimately lead to an increase in vector-borne diseases.

Habitat Changes

An environmental condition that involves a change or modification affecting the livelihood and natural biodiversity in an ecosystem is termed a Habitat change. The effect of climate change alters the habitats of rodents, thus forcing them to move to another suitable environment, where they can carry and spread the pathogen, contributing to disease outbreaks.

Deforestation

Converting the forest lands into agricultural land increased the exposure of rodents to humans. The natural habitat of the rodents living in the jungle is disturbed, and an increase in domestic and peri-domestic rodent exposure has driven many to haphazard behavior, leading to a rise in vector-borne zoonoses and human-animal accidents. Forest fires have forced rodents carrying hundreds of pathogens to enter human dwellings, spreading the disease. A notable example is the KFD, where humans are the accidental dead-end hosts [30].

Urbanization

Population growth and associated overcrowding have contributed to the rise of major communicable diseases, notably upper respiratory tract infections. The practice of poor personal hygiene and sanitation is a significant risk factor for scrub typhus infection. The proper availability of safe drinking water and the equitable distribution of resources are important during disease outbreaks. The lowered GDP (Gross Domestic Product) and GNP (Gross National Product) in poor and developing countries require caution in health beliefs and model development. Urban sewage and sullage plants, as well as their associated drainages and effluents, have created an environment conducive to the growth of rodents that harbor diseases. [38].

Agriculture

The practice of shifting cultivation has led to the migration of humans and rodent populations. Scrub typhus majorly affects agricultural labourers due to their exposure to rodents and bushes. Poor knowledge about the disease and its risk factors is the major reason for the poor to be vulnerable. Different cropping seasons and patterns, such as Kharif and Rabi, are widely practiced in the Southeast Asian regions. Climate change has altered the cultivation and harvesting patterns. Rural inhabitants, who rely on agriculture, can experience heightened human exposure due to increased rainfall. Farmers working in fields and people engaging in outdoor activities, such as collecting firewood, as well as children playing outdoors during or after the monsoon seasons, are at a greater risk of coming into contact with chigger infestations and contracting infections and diseases [23, 39, 40].

Food Patterns

The change in climate affects the food pattern of the rodents. Rodents, such as rats and mice, are typically found in areas like warehouses, godowns, factories, and hotels where large quantities of food are stored. Rodents, when exposed to these food particles, drop their saliva, urine, bites, and other pathogens, which mainly cause food-borne infections like Salmonellosis and other vector-borne diseases, such as leptospirosis, Hantavirus infection, and Scrub typhus, in humans. The presence of moisture and humidity invites numerous disease-transmitting pathogens. Scrub typhus-transmitting rodent reservoirs are found during the wetter seasons, thus increasing the incidence of cases [41, 42].

Disease Transmission

The incubation period for transmission of infection from infected chigger mites to humans is typically 5 to 14 days. Upon invading humans, the bacteria multiply, leading to symptoms such as fever, headache, rash, and in some cases, a characteristic symptom called "Eschar" (a dark, scab-like lesion) at the site of the chigger bite is formed [17, 18].

Rodents carrying Scrub typhus pathogens are primarily found transmitting the disease during the monsoon and post-monsoon seasons, with endemicity throughout the globe. Rodents are carriers of various diseases that can affect humans, such as leptospirosis, Scrub typhus, and plague. The change in climate has led to the emergence of many diseases, with a change in the trend of disease mortality and morbidity.

Ecosystem Impact

The rodents living with a very short life span adapt to the changing environmental patterns. During the evolving era of urbanization, many rodents have become extinct on the islands due to human-made activities, thus predicting the evolutionary outcomes [43]. A study in Texas, using models of vegetation and geography, predicted the impact of climate change on rodent distribution and species composition [44].

Industrialization

The emission of greenhouse gases, such as carbon dioxide, Methane, and Nitrous oxide, has had an impact on climate change, thereby altering the disease pattern. Scrub typhus, previously known to affect rural areas, is now recognized as a global disease, affecting both urban and rural settings. The migration of living beings due to industrialization has enabled the spread of rickettsial infections, namely Scrub Typhus. The proper and timely disposal of biomedical waste from the pharmaceutical industry will help protect humans from rodent-pathogen interactions, thus lowering the risk of contracting occupational infections [45].

Antimicrobial Resistance

The recent advancements in the evolution of Antimicrobial Resistance (AMR) have put a spotlight on society. Doxycycline, a drug of choice for Scrub typhus, has now started developing resistance among patients visiting tertiary care hospitals, as observed in a study carried out in Nepal [1, 46]. The use of combined drugs in cases of Scrub typhus co-infected with other bacterial or viral infections has altered the resistance mechanism, resulting in mutations in the gene sequence. The timely treatment of Scrub typhus will help us avoid antimicrobial resistance.

Disaster Management

The management of Triage during difficult times of disaster plays a pivotal role in controlling disaster mitigation. The unpredictable environmental disasters caused by climate change have presented challenges in controlling vector-borne diseases, namely notifiable diseases, to prevent their spread.

The pre-disaster monitoring and tracking of environmental conditions, such as rainfall, temperature, and rodent populations, before the onset of disaster-prone seasons (monsoons and pre-monsoons), will help predict areas at risk for scrub typhus outbreaks. This enables timely public health responses. Integrated teams, such as Rapid Response Teams, ensure the swift identification of scrub typhus cases and provision of appropriate treatment in disaster-affected areas. The supply of timely medicines, such as antibiotics, doxycycline, and chloramphenicol, should be stockpiled in areas vulnerable to natural disasters, ensuring prompt access to treatment for scrub typhus patients.

In several case studies from the South East Asian region, including South India, which experiences monsoons and frequent flooding, past disasters have often been followed by outbreaks of vector-borne diseases, such as scrub typhus. Epidemiological Studies: Conducting epidemiological studies post-disaster can

help identify specific environmental and social factors that contributed to scrub typhus outbreaks [41, 47 - 50].

LITERATURE SEARCH

A retrospective study on the incidence of Scrub typhus and its correlation with the meteorological factors showed a strong relationship between six meteorological variables: weekly Average Temperature (TEM), weekly Average Relative Humidity (RHU), weekly Average Sunshine Duration (SSD), weekly Average Wind Speed (WIND), weekly Average Pressure (PRS), and weekly Average Precipitation (PRE) with the weekly raise of Scrub typhus cases [51]. Climate change has a significant impact on infectious diseases, such as scrub typhus. The disease is reported as a climate-sensitive rickettsial infection worldwide. The infected chigger mites causing Scrub typhus infection are classified as ectothermic arthropods that are highly climate-dependent. Upon running the Poisson regression model to study the correlation between temperature, Scrub typhus incidence, and precipitation, the results showed a linear relationship [52]. During a seasonal study conducted in South Korea in late summer and autumn to study the relationship between scrub typhus incidence and meteorological factors, the results showed a negative correlation between Scrub incidence and relative humidity [53]. The scrub typhus incidence modeling study carried out in South Korea showed the correlation between Scrub incidences and meteorological factors [15].

Impact on Public Health Interventions

1. **Surveillance and Monitoring**: Understanding the relationship between rainfall and scrub typhus can help public health authorities predict potential outbreaks of scrub typhus. Enhanced surveillance during and after rainy seasons can lead to early detection and prompt response.
2. **Preventive Measures**: During periods of heavy rainfall, communities can be educated about the risks of scrub typhus and the importance of preventive measures, such as avoiding areas with dense vegetation, using insect repellents, and wearing protective clothing.
3. **Environmental Management**: Controlling vegetation around residential areas and eliminating rodent habitats can help reduce the risk of chigger infestations and subsequent transmission of scrub typhus.

Impact on Agriculture and Lifestyle

- **Agriculture:** The monsoon season is crucial for agriculture, as it provides the majority of the annual rainfall required for crops. The timing and intensity of the monsoon can significantly affect agricultural productivity. The peri-domestic rodents in the agricultural lands near the sea.
- **Lifestyle:** Seasonal changes significantly impact daily life, including clothing, diet, and festivals. For instance, winter is a popular season for weddings and festivals, while summer heat drives people to seek cooler climates or stay indoors.

People Vulnerable to Scrub Typhus

Dating back to the history of war in 1947, Scrub typhus was found to be more common among soldiers who were often exposed to forests and trekking [38].

Developing countries like India, with falling GDPs, produce a miserable life for the poor portion of the population, making them more vulnerable and susceptible to communicable and non-communicable diseases. The vector-borne zoonosis, namely Anthropozoonoses, including rickettsial infections, Such as Scrub typhus, is more prevalent, as evident in the literature, with a prevalence of approximately 20.2%. The disease remains mainly underdiagnosed and underreported, often presenting as Fever of Unknown Origin (FUO) or Pyrexia of Unknown Origin (PUO). The regions endemic to Scrub typhus were those where agriculture was the main occupation, with the rural population being more exposed. Farmers working in agricultural fields with limited knowledge of hygiene and sanitation, walking barefoot, taking naps under trees without a mat, and not practicing the habit of bathing and hand-washing techniques have made them more susceptible to rodent exposure, thus becoming accidental hosts. The gender bias of the disease shows that males are more susceptible hosts to Scrub typhus than females.

Protective Measures

- The root control of Scrub typhus involves vector control measures, such as the use of rodenticides to control the rodent population.
- Self-care measures, such as adopting a habit of personal hygiene and sanitation, as well as wearing sleeve dresses and boots when exploring bushy areas, can reduce exposure to rodent-borne diseases.
- The timely diagnosis of the clinical signs and symptoms of Scrub typhus, such as the presence of Eschar in hidden areas, is mandatory for early treatment and recovery from the disease, thereby reducing mortality and morbidity.
- An antibiotic, "Tetracycline," which is the drug of choice, is to be administered timely for early recovery.
- Washing hands with soap and maintaining personal hygiene.
- Using insect repellents with DEET to avoid mosquito and tick bites. Use pyrethrum-treated clothes and bed nets if necessary. Integrated pest management plays a vital role.
- Review the patient's medical history thoroughly for the presence of hidden Eschar and rashes.
- Purchase evacuation insurance, register with the local embassy, and familiarize yourself with evacuation procedures before ascent.

Role of Public Health Professionals

According to Bloom's taxonomy, learning begins with knowledge, and this knowledge must be disseminated to the population through social public health activists. The use of mass communication through the media helps reach the message to a larger audience. The health-for-all approach delivers the equitable distribution of resources. Health professionals play a crucial role in the prevention, diagnosis, and management of scrub typhus:

Primary care workers and grassroots-level workers, such as ASHA (Accredited Social Health Activists), play a frontline defense role in controlling vector-borne diseases, especially during disease outbreaks [54]. Community health care workers at the Primary and Community Health Centres are public health professionals whose major role is to bring people suspected of having Scrub typhus to the healthcare centres and provide them with timely diagnosis and treatment. The BCC (Behaviour Change Communication) must be effectively implemented in the community to educate the public about the risk factors associated with the disease and the seriousness of its aftereffects. The ANMs (Auxiliary Nurse Midwives) and lab technicians must be pre-qualified to carry out laboratory tests and generate reports in a timely manner.

The disease is often misdiagnosed with other Fever of Unknown Origin (FUO), making it a herculean task for health professionals to diagnose the disease. During outbreaks, frontline workers and healthcare experts must verify the outbreak, confirm it with lab reports, and contain the zones in case of contagious diseases.

In summary, health professionals at all levels—from community nurses to infectious disease experts—need to collaborate to raise awareness, enhance diagnosis, and provide timely and appropriate management of scrub typhus. Strengthening the healthcare system's capacity is crucial to tackling this emerging public health threat.

Role of the Government

The government must strictly adhere to laws and regulations by implementing new policies at the state and district level authorities, thus decentralizing power.

1. National Centre for Disease Control (NCDC) Programs

The **NCDC**, under the Ministry of Health and Family Welfare (MoHFW), plays a critical role in controlling vector-borne diseases, including scrub typhus. The NCDC has undertaken several actions such as:

- **Surveillance and Monitoring**: NCDC monitors scrub typhus cases through its Integrated Disease Surveillance Programme (IDSP). It collects data on scrub typhus outbreaks, helping in early detection and response.
- **Guidelines and Protocols**: The NCDC has issued guidelines for the diagnosis, treatment, and management of scrub typhus. These guidelines are distributed to healthcare providers nationwide, ensuring standardized care.

- **Training and Capacity Building**: The NCDC regularly conducts training for healthcare professionals on the identification and treatment of scrub typhus. They aim to enhance diagnostic capabilities, especially in rural and endemic areas.

2. Integrated Disease Surveillance Programme (IDSP)

The **IDSP** is a major initiative by the Indian government aimed at strengthening disease surveillance nationwide. Scrub typhus is one of the diseases included in this program.

- **Surveillance Data**: The IDSP collects real-time data on scrub typhus cases across India, enabling prompt responses to outbreaks and informing public health strategies.
- **Outbreak Response**: In the event of scrub typhus outbreaks, the IDSP coordinates with state health departments to implement containment measures, including vector control and public awareness campaigns.

3. National Vector Borne Disease Control Programme (NVBDCP)

The **NVBDCP** is another important program under the Ministry of Health and Family Welfare, primarily focused on vector-borne diseases such as malaria and dengue, but it also covers diseases transmitted by mites, including scrub typhus [55].

- **Integrated Vector Management (IVM)**: The NVBDCP promotes vector control strategies that include the management of chigger mites (larval mites that spread scrub typhus) through environmental measures such as rodent control, cleaning up areas prone to infestation, and reducing mite breeding grounds.

4. Health Education and Public Awareness Campaigns

Government agencies, particularly at the state level, run public awareness campaigns aimed at educating people in endemic areas about the prevention of scrub typhus. These campaigns focus on:

- Promoting personal protective measures, such as using insect repellents and wearing protective clothing when working in fields.
- Raising awareness about the importance of early diagnosis and treatment, particularly in rural areas where access to healthcare may be limited.

5. State-Specific Programs

Certain Indian states where scrub typhus is endemic, such as Tamil Nadu, Kerala, Himachal Pradesh, and Uttarakhand, have developed state-specific strategies. These strategies often include:

- **Enhanced Surveillance**: States actively collect data on scrub typhus cases and identify hot spots for targeted interventions.
- **Free Treatment Programs**: Some states provide free treatment for scrub typhus at government health centers.
- **Special Task Forces**: In states like Kerala, task forces have been created to address vector-borne diseases, including scrub typhus. These task forces coordinate with local health workers to detect and treat cases early.

6. Collaborations with International Organizations

The Indian government frequently collaborates with international health organizations, such as the World Health Organization (WHO) and the Centers for Disease Control and Prevention (CDC), for capacity building, research, and control measures against scrub typhus and other vector-borne diseases [56].

- **WHO's Southeast Asia Regional Office (SEARO)** provides technical support for surveillance, diagnostics, and outbreak response.
- **CDC Collaborations**: The CDC has collaborated with Indian health authorities to enhance laboratory capacity for diagnosing scrub typhus, improve reporting systems, and research effective control measures.

7. Research and Development Initiatives

Government research bodies, such as the Indian Council of Medical Research (ICMR), are actively engaged in research on scrub typhus. Their initiatives include:

- Studying the epidemiology of scrub typhus to understand its distribution and risk factors.
- Developing diagnostic tools that are more affordable and accessible for use in rural health centers.
- Research on vaccines and treatment protocols to improve disease management.

8. Rodent Control and Environmental Management Programs

Since rodents are key reservoirs of scrub typhus, rodent control measures are often part of broader environmental management programs implemented by local governments. These programs may involve:

- Cleaning up rodent-infested areas, especially in farming or forested regions.
- Educating farmers on practices that can reduce the risk of rodent and mite infestations, such as proper storage of food and agricultural products.
- Encouraging sanitation measures to reduce rodent populations in human habitats.

Controlling Climate Change

The acceleration of the Sustainable Development Goals (SDGs) plays a crucial role in achieving the 3rd and 13th goals, specifically "Good health and wellbeing" and "Climate Action."

Infrastructure: Building infrastructure that can withstand extreme weather events and sea-level rise. The use of advanced technologies to overcome disaster mitigation.

Agricultural Practices: Developing drought-resistant crops and improving water management helps overcome scarcity during disasters.

Disaster Preparedness: Enhancing early warning systems and emergency response plans to escape from the disaster.

Policy and International Cooperation:

Paris Agreement: A legally binding global climate change agreement, the Paris Agreement was ratified by 196 nations in 2015. The agreement's main objectives are to hold the increase in the global average temperature to well below 2 °C above pre-industrial levels and to pursue efforts to restrict it to 1.5°C. Additionally, it aims to coordinate financial flows to promote growth that is climate-resilient and emits fewer greenhouse gases. Nationally Determined Contributions (NDCs), or country-specific climate action plans, must be established and regularly updated by each member of the agreement. Notwithstanding their lack of legal force, the NDCs provide a platform for openness, responsibility, and forward-thinking climate action. In 2016, the Paris Agreement came into effect after receiving enough ratifications from nations. Courts are utilizing their objectives to rule against governments and corporations for not doing enough to address climate change, and it has become a focal point for climate change litigation. All things considered, the Paris Agreement represents a historic global effort to mitigate climate change and its impacts. Although its efficacy is still up for discussion, it has spurred international action and cooperation.

Public Awareness and Education

The World Health Organisation (WHO), along with organizations like UNICEF (United Nations International Children's Emergency Fund), SIDA (Swedish International Development Cooperation Agency), DANIDA (Danish International Development Agency), the Indian Red Cross, and Bill and Melinda Gates have been vigorously working against the communicable and non communicable control of diseases.

Early Diagnosis and Complete Treatment (EDCT)

The program focuses on early diagnosis and timely treatment of scrub typhus to reduce mortality and morbidity associated with the disease. Due to the evolving strategies of disease detection and treatment, the disease has now become a focus of attention for the nation, with differential diagnostic techniques being implemented to diagnose Scrub typhus using both serological and molecular assays. The ancient technique of the Weil-Felix test, which has low sensitivity and specificity, requires no skilled laborers. The use of ELISA tests to detect IgM and IgG antibodies with high sensitivity and specificity is widely used in public laboratories. The molecular assay targeting antigens through PCR sequencing is the best method for identifying serotypic strains circulating in the region. Doxycycline is a suitable drug of choice that should be administered to the patient immediately after receiving positive lab results. The intravenous administration of doxycycline during severe conditions will lower the mortality rate and increase the recovery rate. The use of combination drug therapy in cases of co-infections plays a significant role in disease control mechanisms.

One Health Approach

Bringing together the concern of the epidemiological triad, the one health approach seeks to involve all components of this interconnected triangle, whose control will help us control disease transmission. Various interconnected climate change activities, such as seminars, symposia, and conferences, have made us aware of the effectiveness of the one health approach. The inputs of the expert commission groups in implementing the program strategies have resulted in great control of vector-borne disease transmission. Several health policies are demonstrating high efficacy in reducing disease transmission.

Educating communities about risk factors for scrub typhus, including rodent control, personal protective measures, and environmental management, will help reduce exposure of rodents to humans. The training of healthcare workers to recognize scrub typhus symptoms, especially in endemic areas like Thiruvarur, and promoting early treatment with appropriate antibiotics (like doxycycline) is crucial for reducing mortality [57].

Early monitoring of human health, rodent populations, and environmental conditions helps identify early signs and symptoms of potential outbreaks. The advancement in utilizing Geographic Information Systems (GIS) to map cases of scrub typhus alongside rodent population data and environmental changes (*e.g.*, rainfall, deforestation) can help identify hotspots for targeted interventions. An integrated approach to one health is a key to preventing vector-borne diseases.

Recent Data on Scrub Typhus

Deforestation and urbanization have evolved into scrub typhus outbreaks with a changing epidemiology of the agent, host, and environment. Human exposure to forest areas and agricultural-related occupations are more prone to scrub typhus since rodents and vector mites are in close proximity to humans, thus making humans accidental hosts. The cases are more prevalent in urbanized areas of tropical and subtropical regions.

The changing dynamics of scrub typhus across the globe are marked by skepticism regarding case outbreaks. The changing effects of meteorological factors on scrub typhus cases in China from 2010 to 2019 resulted in 9,034 scrub typhus cases, with an annual rise in cases from 8.49 to 62.96 per 100,000, peaking in August. Also, Thailand reported 31 cases of Scrub typhus from June 2018 and December 2019 [58].

Mathematical Model on Scrub Typhus

The mathematical models would help predict the transmission of disease based on the current incidence of the disease. These models will help disease-endemic areas to be cautious about future outbreaks and how to tackle and manage their severity. The use of the basic reproduction number (R_0) in mathematical models indicates the secondary cases that arise from a single infected person in the susceptible population. The models will help us in the following ways;

1. Risk assessment and control measures
2. Policy Planning and Management
3. Data interpretation

4. Disease severity
5. Disease mitigation

CONCLUSION

Scrub typhus, a vector-borne zoonotic infection, has shown a proportionate trend of change in incidence with changing environmental patterns. The effects of temperature, humidity, and rainfall play a pivotal role in cases of scrub typhus. The evolving research on climate change and vector-borne diseases is an important topic to be discussed and covered under the one health approach.

Scrub typhus, a vector borne disease transmitted by chigger mites, is intricately linked to environmental factors, making it vulnerable to the effects of **climate change**. As climate patterns shift, particularly through changes in temperature, rainfall, and humidity, the dynamics of scrub typhus transmission are likely to change as well. The increasing frequency of extreme weather events, such as floods, and rising temperatures contribute to favorable conditions for rodent and mite populations, which are the key reservoirs and vectors of the disease.

1. **Increased Transmission Risk**: Climate change may lead to more frequent and severe scrub typhus outbreaks by expanding suitable habitats for chiggers and rodents, especially in regions with altered rainfall patterns or warming temperatures. Regions that were previously unaffected may become new hot spots for the disease.
2. **Seasonal Shifts**: With altered climate patterns, the transmission seasons for scrub typhus may shift or extend, leading to changes in the timing of disease outbreaks. In areas where monsoon seasons become more intense or prolonged, the post-monsoon period may see an increase in cases due to increased vegetation, rodent populations, and human exposure.
3. **Environmental Disturbances**: Deforestation, urbanization, and agricultural expansion, driven in part by climate pressures, may push rodents closer to human habitats, increasing the risk of human contact with infected mites. Natural disasters, such as floods and landslides, exacerbated by climate change, can also drive rodents into human settlements, increasing the potential for disease transmission.
4. **Challenges for Public Health Systems**: Climate change complicates the control of scrub typhus by creating unpredictable transmission patterns. Public health systems will need to be agile, with enhanced surveillance, early detection, and response mechanisms, especially in rural and forested areas where the disease is most prevalent.

REFERENCES

[1] Dhiman RC, Pahwa S, Dhillon GPS, Dash AP. Climate change and threat of vector-borne diseases in India: are we prepared? Parasitol Res 2010; 106(4): 763-73.
[http://dx.doi.org/10.1007/s00436-010-1767-4] [PMID: 20155369]

[2] Semenza JC, Rocklöv J, Ebi KL. Climate change and cascading risks from infectious disease. Infect Dis Ther 2022; 11(4): 1371-90.
[http://dx.doi.org/10.1007/s40121-022-00647-3] [PMID: 35585385]

[3] Vonesch N, D'Ovidio MC, Melis P, Remoli ME, Ciufolini MG, Tomao P. Climate change, vector-borne diseases and working population. Ann Ist Super Sanita 2016; 52(3): 397-405.
[PMID: 27698298]

[4] Sadanandane C, Jambulingam P, Paily KP, *et al.* Occurrence of *Orientia tsutsugamushi*, the etiological agent of scrub typhus in animal hosts and mite vectors in areas reporting human cases of acute encephalitis syndrome in the gorakhpur region of Uttar Pradesh, India. Vector Borne Zoonotic Dis 2018; 18(10): 539-47.
[http://dx.doi.org/10.1089/vbz.2017.2246] [PMID: 30016222]

[5] Tantibhedhyangkul W, Ben Amara A, Textoris J, *et al.* Orientia tsutsugamushi, the causative agent of scrub typhus, induces an inflammatory program in human macrophages. Microb Pathog 2013; 55: 55-63.
[http://dx.doi.org/10.1016/j.micpath.2012.10.001] [PMID: 23088884]

[6] Kuo CC, Lee PL, Chen CH, Wang HC. Surveillance of potential hosts and vectors of scrub typhus in Taiwan. Parasit Vectors 2015; 8(1): 611.
[http://dx.doi.org/10.1186/s13071-015-1221-7] [PMID: 26626287]

[7] Elliott I, Pearson I, Dahal P, Thomas NV, Roberts T, Newton PN. Scrub typhus ecology: a systematic review of Orientia in vectors and hosts. Parasit Vectors 2019; 12(1): 513.
[http://dx.doi.org/10.1186/s13071-019-3751-x] [PMID: 31685019]

[8] Devaraju P, Arumugam B, Mohan I, *et al.* Evidence of natural infection of *Orientia tsutsugamushi* in vectors and animal hosts – Risk of scrub typhus transmission to humans in Puducherry, South India. Indian J Public Health 2020; 64(1): 27-31.
[http://dx.doi.org/10.4103/ijph.IJPH_130_19] [PMID: 32189679]

[9] Tanskul P, Strickman D, Eamsila C, Kelly DJ. Rickettsia tsutsugamushi in chiggers (Acari: Trombiculidae) associated with rodents in central Thailand. J Med Entomol 1994; 31(2): 225-30.
[http://dx.doi.org/10.1093/jmedent/31.2.225] [PMID: 8189414]

[10] Akhunji B, Bhate R, Pansare N, *et al.* Distribution of Orientia tsutsugamushi in rodents and mites collected from Central India. Environ Monit Assess 2019; 191(2): 82.
[http://dx.doi.org/10.1007/s10661-019-7208-7] [PMID: 30656500]

[11] Candasamy S, Ayyanar E, Paily K, Karthikeyan PA, Sundararajan A, Purushothaman J. Abundance & distribution of trombiculid mites & *Orientia tsutsugamushi*, the vectors & pathogen of scrub typhus in rodents & shrews collected from Puducherry & Tamil Nadu, India. Indian J Med Res 2016; 144(6): 893-900.
[http://dx.doi.org/10.4103/ijmr.IJMR_1390_15] [PMID: 28474626]

[12] Zangpo T, Phuentshok Y, Dorji K, *et al.* Environmental, occupational, and demographic risk factors for clinical scrub typhus, Bhutan. Emerg Infect Dis 2023; 29(5): 909-18.
[http://dx.doi.org/10.3201/eid2905.221430] [PMID: 37081000]

[13] Mohapatra R K, Al-Haideri M, Mishra S, *et al.* Linking the increasing epidemiology of scrub typhus transmission in India and South Asia: are the varying environment and the reservoir animals the factors behind? Front Trop Dis 2024; 5

[14] Kwak J, Kim S, Kim G, Singh V, Hong S, Kim H. Scrub typhus incidence modeling with meteorological factors in South Korea. Int J Environ Res Public Health 2015; 12(7): 7254-73.

[http://dx.doi.org/10.3390/ijerph120707254] [PMID: 26132479]

[15]   Eldin C, Parola P. Rickettsioses as causes of CNS infection in southeast Asia. Lancet Glob Health 2015; 3(2): e67-8.
[http://dx.doi.org/10.1016/S2214-109X(14)70379-1] [PMID: 25617194]

[16]   Lee SH, Lee YS, Lee IY, *et al.* Monthly occurrence of vectors and reservoir rodents of scrub typhus in an endemic area of Jeollanam-do, Korea. Korean J Parasitol 2012; 50(4): 327-31.
[http://dx.doi.org/10.3347/kjp.2012.50.4.327] [PMID: 23230330]

[17]   Paris DH, Phetsouvanh R, Tanganuchitcharnchai A, *et al.* Orientia tsutsugamushi in human scrub typhus eschars shows tropism for dendritic cells and monocytes rather than endothelium. PLoS Negl Trop Dis 2012; 6(1): e1466.
[http://dx.doi.org/10.1371/journal.pntd.0001466] [PMID: 22253938]

[18]   Win AM, Nguyen YTH, Kim Y, *et al.* Genotypic heterogeneity of *Orientia tsutsugamushi* in scrub typhus patients and thrombocytopenia syndrome co-infection, Myanmar. Emerg Infect Dis 2020; 26(8): 1878-81.
[http://dx.doi.org/10.3201/eid2608.200135] [PMID: 32687023]

[19]   Samuel PP, Govindarajan R, Rajamannar V, Kumar A. Current status of mites and mite-borne diseases in India. J Vector Borne Dis 2023; 60(1): 1-10.
[http://dx.doi.org/10.4103/0972-9062.361175] [PMID: 37026214]

[20]   Chaisiri K, Tanganuchitcharnchai A, Kritiyakan A, *et al.* Risk factors analysis for neglected human rickettsioses in rural communities in Nan province, Thailand: A community-based observational study along a landscape gradient. PLoS Negl Trop Dis 2022; 16(3): e0010256.
[http://dx.doi.org/10.1371/journal.pntd.0010256] [PMID: 35320277]

[21]   Govindarajan R, Rajamannar V, Krishnamoorthi R, Kumar A, Samuel PP. Distribution pattern of chigger mites in south Tamil Nadu, India. Entomon 2021; 46(3): 247-54.
[http://dx.doi.org/10.33307/entomon.v46i3.611]

[22]   Santibáñez P, Palomar AM, Portillo A, Santibáñez S, Oteo JA. The role of chiggers as human pathogens. An Overview of Tropical Diseases. 2015.
[http://dx.doi.org/10.5772/61978]

[23]   Pan K, Huang R, Xu L, Lin F. Exploring the effects and interactions of meteorological factors on the incidence of scrub typhus in Ganzhou City, 2008–2021. BMC Public Health 2024; 24(1): 36.
[http://dx.doi.org/10.1186/s12889-023-17423-8] [PMID: 38167033]

[24]   Rajapakse S, Rodrigo C. Treatment of dengue fever. Infect Drug Resist 2012; 103.

[25]   PicKard AL, McDaniel P, Miller RS, *et al.* A study of febrile illnesses on the Thai-Myanmar border: predictive factors of rickettsioses. Southeast Asian J Trop Med Public Health 2004; 35(3): 657-63.
[PMID: 15689083]

[26]   Xiang J, Hansen A, Liu Q, *et al.* Association between dengue fever incidence and meteorological factors in Guangzhou, China, 2005–2014. Environ Res 2017; 153: 17-26.
[http://dx.doi.org/10.1016/j.envres.2016.11.009] [PMID: 27883970]

[27]   Matsumura Y, Shimizu T. Case of imported scrub typhus contracted in Myanmar. Kansenshogaku Zasshi 2009; 83(3): 256-60.
[http://dx.doi.org/10.11150/kansenshogakuzasshi.83.256] [PMID: 19522310]

[28]   Kumar Bhat N, Dhar M, Mittal G, *et al.* Scrub typhus in children at a tertiary hospital in north India: clinical profile and complications. Iran J Pediatr 2014; 24(4): 387-92.
[PMID: 25755859]

[29]   Sharma Parag, Kakkar Rakesh. Geographical distribution, effect of season & life cycle of scrub typhus. JK Sci J Med Edu Res 2010; 63-4.

[30]   Krishnan J, Shukla A, Rajalakshmi A, *et al.* Seasonal variations of dengue vector mosquitoes in rural

settings of Thiruvarur district in Tamil Nadu, India. J Vector Borne Dis 2020; 57(1): 63-70.
[http://dx.doi.org/10.4103/0972-9062.308803] [PMID: 33818458]

[31] Mogi M. Relationship between number of human Japanese encephalitis cases and summer meteorological conditions in Nagasaki, Japan. Am J Trop Med Hyg 1983; 32(1): 170-4.
[http://dx.doi.org/10.4269/ajtmh.1983.32.170] [PMID: 6297324]

[32] Tilak R, Kunte R. Scrub typhus strikes back: Are we ready? Med J Armed Forces India 2019; 75(1): 8-17.
[http://dx.doi.org/10.1016/j.mjafi.2018.12.018] [PMID: 30705472]

[33] D'Cruz S, Sreedevi K, Lynette C, Gunasekaran K, Prakash JAJ. Climate influences scrub typhus occurrence in Vellore, Tamil Nadu, India: analysis of a 15-year dataset. Sci Rep 2024; 14(1): 1532.
[http://dx.doi.org/10.1038/s41598-023-49333-5] [PMID: 38233417]

[34] Sharma AK. Eco-entomological investigation in Scrub Typhus affected area of Thiruvananthapuram, Kerala (India) and their control/containment measures. Int J Curr Microbiol Appl Sci 2013.

[35] Dasgupta S, Asish PR, Rachel G, Bagepally BS, Chethrapilly Purushothaman GK. Global seroprevalence of scrub typhus: a systematic review and meta-analysis. Sci Rep 2024; 14(1): 10895.
[http://dx.doi.org/10.1038/s41598-024-61555-9] [PMID: 38740885]

[36] Basnyat B, Cumbo T A, Edelman R. Infections at high altitude 2001; 33(11)
[http://dx.doi.org/10.1086/324163]

[37] Park JW, Yu DS, Lee GS, Seo JJ, Chung JK, Lee JI. Il. Epidemiological characteristics of rodents and chiggers with orientia tsutsugamushi in the republic of Korea. Korean J Parasitol 2020; 58(5): 559-64.
[http://dx.doi.org/10.3347/kjp.2020.58.5.559] [PMID: 33202508]

[38] Premaratna R. Rickettsial illnesses, a leading cause of acute febrile illness. Clin Med (Lond) 2022; 22(1): 2-5.
[http://dx.doi.org/10.7861/clinmed.2021-0790] [PMID: 35078787]

[39] Ramasamy R, Surendran SN. Global climate change and its potential impact on disease transmission by salinity-tolerant mosquito vectors in coastal zones. JUN, Frontiers in Physiology 2012; Vol. 3.

[40] Singh SI, Devi KP, Tilotama R, *et al.* An outbreak of scrub typhus in Bishnupur district of Manipur, India, 2007. Trop Doct 2010; 40(3): 169-70.
[http://dx.doi.org/10.1258/td.2010.090468] [PMID: 20555047]

[41] Richards AL, Soeatmadji DW, Widodo MA, *et al.* Seroepidemiologic evidence for murine and scrub typhus in Malang, Indonesia. Am J Trop Med Hyg 1997; 57(1): 91-5.
[http://dx.doi.org/10.4269/ajtmh.1997.57.91] [PMID: 9242326]

[42] Auffray J-C, Claude J. Rodent Biodiversity in Changing Environments SEE PROFILE 2009.

[43] Cameron GN, Scheel D. Getting warmer: effect of global climate change on distribution of rodents in Texas. J Mammal. 2001; 82.(3)

[44] Lokida D, Hadi U, Lau CY, *et al.* Underdiagnoses of Rickettsia in patients hospitalized with acute fever in Indonesia: observational study results. BMC Infect Dis 2020; 20(1): 364.
[http://dx.doi.org/10.1186/s12879-020-05057-9] [PMID: 32448167]

[45] Dhiman RC, Pahwa S, Dhillon GPS, Dash AP. Climate change and threat of vector-borne diseases in India: are we prepared? Parasitol Res. 2010; 106: pp. (4)763-73.

[46] Vivekanandan M, Mani A, Priya YS, Singh AP, Jayakumar S, Purty S. Outbreak of scrub typhus in Pondicherry. J Assoc Physicians India 2010; 58(1): 24-8.
[PMID: 20649095]

[47] Swain SK, Sahu BP, Panda S, Sarangi R, Sarangi R. Molecular characterization and evolutionary analysis of Orientia tsutsugamushi in eastern Indian population. Arch Microbiol 2022; 204(4): 221.
[http://dx.doi.org/10.1007/s00203-022-02823-y] [PMID: 35338394]

[48]   Sinha P, Gupta S, Dawra R, Rijhawan P. Recent outbreak of scrub typhus in North Western part of India. Indian J Med Microbiol 2014; 32(3): 247-50.
[http://dx.doi.org/10.4103/0255-0857.136552] [PMID: 25008815]

[49]   Mathai E, Rolain JM, Verghese GM, *et al.* Outbreak of scrub typhus in southern India during the cooler months. Ann N Y Acad Sci 2003; 990(1): 359-64.
[http://dx.doi.org/10.1111/j.1749-6632.2003.tb07391.x] [PMID: 12860654]

[50]   Ma CJ, Oh GJ, Kang GU, *et al.* Differences in agricultural activities related to incidence of scrub typhus between Korea and Japan. Epidemiol Health 2017; 39: e2017051.
[http://dx.doi.org/10.4178/epih.e2017051] [PMID: 29121711]

[51]   Li W, Niu Y, Ren H, *et al.* Climate-driven scrub typhus incidence dynamics in South China: A time-series study. Front Environ Sci 2022; 10: 849681.
[http://dx.doi.org/10.3389/fenvs.2022.849681]

[52]   Kim YJ, Park S, Premaratna R, *et al.* Clinical evaluation of rapid diagnostic test kit for scrub typhus with improved performance. J Korean Med Sci 2016; 31(8): 1190-6.
[http://dx.doi.org/10.3346/jkms.2016.31.8.1190] [PMID: 27478327]

[53]   Koralur M, Singh R, Varma M, *et al.* Scrub typhus diagnosis on acute specimens using serological and molecular assays — a 3-year prospective study. Diagn Microbiol Infect Dis 2018; 91(2): 112-7.
[http://dx.doi.org/10.1016/j.diagmicrobio.2018.01.018] [PMID: 29706479]

[54]   WHO. A global brief on vector-borne diseases. World Health Organization 2014.

[55]   Guidelines for Diagnosis, Treatment, Prevention and Control. WHO Regional Publication SEARO 2009; 2009: 1-144.

[56]   Rahi M, Gupte MD, Bhargava A, Varghese G, Arora R. DHR-ICMR Guidelines for diagnosis & management of Rickettsial diseases in India. Indian J Med Res 2015; 141(4): 417-22.
[http://dx.doi.org/10.4103/0971-5916.159279] [PMID: 26112842]

[57]   Faburay B. The case for a 'one health' approach to combating vector-borne diseases. Infect Ecol Epidemiol 2015; 5(1): 28132.
[http://dx.doi.org/10.3402/iee.v5.28132] [PMID: 26027713]

[58]   Adhikari P, Shrestha A, Donovan SM, Koirala J. Editorial: Scrub typhus & its changing dynamics. Frontiers in Tropical Diseases 2024; 5: 1511950.
[http://dx.doi.org/10.3389/fitd.2024.1511950]

CHAPTER 3

Climate Change and Kyasanur Forest Disease (KFD)

Sathya Jeevitha Balakrishnan[1] and Jayalakshmi Krishnan[1,*]

[1] *Vector Biology Research Laboratory, Department of Biotechnology, Central University of Tamil Nadu, Thiruvarur, India*

Abstract: Climate change is significantly impacting the epidemiology of Kyasanur Forest Disease [KFD], a viral tick-borne hemorrhagic fever indigenous to India's Western Ghats area. Alterations in temperature and precipitation patterns directly affect the survival, development, and activity of *Haemaphysalis spinigera*, the primary vector for KFDV, as well as the distribution and behavior of animal hosts. Warmer and more humid conditions, driven by climate change, create favorable environments for tick proliferation, potentially expanding their geographical range and increasing human-tick interactions. Deforestation and habitat fragmentation also exacerbate the situation by disrupting the balance between vectors, hosts, and humans. This environmental degradation forces animal reservoirs, such as monkeys, and human populations into closer touch, heightening the risk of virus transmission. Seasonal variations play a crucial role, with KFD incidence peaking during the drier, hotter months when tick activity is at its highest. The annual transmission cycle in regions like Shivamogga district shows cases emerging in January, peaking in March, and declining by June, with a resurgence in November, demonstrating a clear link between climate patterns and disease spread. Understanding the intricate relationship between climate change, tick ecology, and KFD transmission is essential for developing effective public health strategies and alleviating future outbreaks. This chapter underscores the urgent need for integrated approaches to address the complex interplay of environmental changes and disease dynamics.

Keywords: Climate change, Diapause, *Haemaphysalis spinigera*, Kyasanur forest disease, Precipitation patterns, Tick.

INTRODUCTION

One of the significant public health and global disease concerns is the vector-borne zoonotic illness that accounts for a larger impact of over 17% of all infectious diseases, including about 700,000 deaths annually. These diseases are

---
* **Corresponding author Jayalakshmi Krishnan:** Vector Biology Research Laboratory, Department of Biotechnology, Central University of Tamil Nadu, Thiruvarur, India; E-mail: jayalakshmi@cutn.ac.in

Jayalakshmi Krishnan, Sigamani Panneer, P. Thiyagarajan, Balachandar Vellingiri & Pradeep Kumar Srivastava (Eds.)

highly transmissible with the help of vectors, such as mosquitoes, mites, fleas, and ticks, which can gather pathogens from infected hosts and transmit them to new hosts. About 75 percent of infectious diseases are zoonotic as they possess the potential for widespread transmission, severe health consequences, and economic impact. Complex factors, including global travel and trade, unplanned urbanization, and environmental changes, drive the emergence and spread of vector-borne diseases. Many zoonotic diseases have serious human health and economic consequences, especially in developing countries with poor diagnostic facilities, lack of medical services, and inadequate hygiene practices [1]. The probability of emerging zoonotic diseases increases with the growing volume of animal trade. Addressing the threat of vector-borne and zoonotic diseases requires a multifaceted approach, including strengthening vector control, improving disease surveillance, reporting, and advancing research on disease ecology, epidemiology, and control strategies. Collaboration between public health agencies, clinicians, and disease ecologists is crucial for early detection and effective management of these emerging health threats. The interaction between human activities and wildlife habitats, coupled with changes in environmental conditions, can increase the likelihood of zoonotic disease outbreaks [2].

One of the most significant vectors for zoonotic illness is ticks, mainly because they are capable of transmitting protozoa, bacteria, and viruses. They transmit critical zoonotic illnesses like Lyme disease, babesiosis, tick-borne encephalitis, anaplasmosis, Kyasanur forest disease, *etc*. Their ability to carry multiple pathogens simultaneously, known as co-infection, can complicate the diagnosis and treatment of tick-borne diseases in humans and animals. They are recognized as the most prevalent ectoparasites that live outside of animals and require feeding on their blood to survive. Recently, the number of recorded instances has increased, with ticks spreading globally and expanding into new regions. These arachnids serve as vectors for various rickettsial and viral diseases. As their bites are undetectable, people often do not even realize they have been bitten in many cases. There are already over 800 species of ticks known to exist, categorized into three families: Argasidae, Ixodidae, and Nuttalliellidae. Climate and environmental factors considerably impact tick dispersion and the diseases they carry. Various factors, including biotic and abiotic elements, the optimal climate for each tick species, and the relationships that ticks have with the diseases they carry are essential to understanding the tick population's global distribution. The worldwide increase in Tick-Borne Diseases [TBDs] is associated with expanding tick habitats, including woody areas, plains, and fields. Furthermore, human activities, such as leaning on logs in parks or resting near trees in tick-containment areas, heighten the possibility of acquiring these infections [3].

Despite widespread tick control methods and advancements in diagnosing Tick-Borne Diseases [TBDs], their numbers are rising globally, with an annual incidence of 50,000 human-reported cases in Europe caused by *Ixodes ricinus*. Chemical options for controlling and managing these diseases may not be enough. A more comprehensive approach is needed to combine chemical control with natural predators, such as spiders, for integrated pest control and improved diagnostics. Additionally, continuous research is crucial for understanding the diverse TBD landscape worldwide [4].

Climate change is exacerbating the spread and transmission of tick-borne diseases like Lyme disease, Kyasanur forest disease, *etc.*, and creating more favorable conditions for tick populations to thrive and expand their geographic range. The two most important climatic factors influencing the regional distribution and abundance of tick species are climate change-related changes in precipitation patterns and warmer temperatures. Milder winters and longer spring and fall seasons enable ticks to be active for a greater portion of the year, allowing them to breed more successfully. Studies have found that the average temperature, diurnal temperature range, and precipitation levels of the hottest quarter are the most important predictors of tick establishment in new areas. Ticks thrive in areas with temperatures above 45°F and at least 85% humidity. As the climate changes, ticks are expanding their range northward by 35-55 km per year in North America and to higher altitudes in Europe. This increases the potential risk of tick-borne illnesses in previously barren areas for ticks [5].

Kyasanur Forest Disease [KFD] is a flaviviral illness that is tick-borne and caused by the Kyasanur Forest Disease Virus [KFDV] that has been rapidly expanding along the Western Ghats, particularly affecting the southern states of India, specifically Karnataka, Kerala, Goa, and Maharashtra. First identified in India in 1957, it is transmitted by infected *Haemaphysalis spinigera* ticks. This virus, belonging to the Flaviviridae family, causes symptoms like high fever, headaches, and bleeding within 3-8 days of infection [6] (Fig. **1**).

Climate change influences temperatures to rise and precipitation patterns to alter, making it easier for the tick vectors that spread KFD to thrive. Research has identified that the typical warmth during the warmest quarter, daily temperature variations, and precipitation levels significantly influence the allocation of *Haemaphysalis spinigera*, the primary tick vector for KFD. Insufficient rainfall and extreme heat in southern India create optimal conditions for tick survival and proliferation. The KFD transmission spans from the month of November to May, when overall total precipitation is less than 500 mm, while heavy rainfall from the month of June to October establishes a conducive ecology for the tick vector. Deforestation and changes in land use have also increased the proximity of the

KFD virus and its carriers to human populations. As climate change progresses, the potential risk areas for KFD are expected to widen, highlighting the necessity for enhanced surveillance and preparedness in currently unaffected regions.

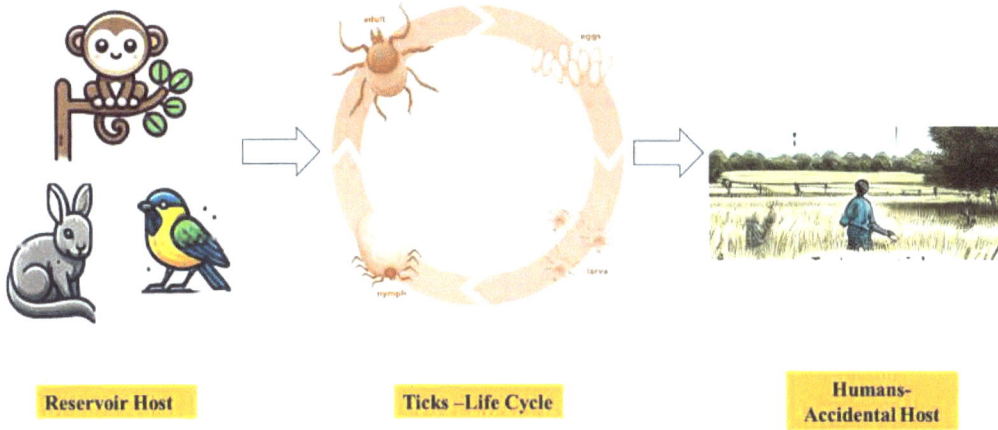

Fig. (1). Transmission dynamics of KFD.

However, climate change is just one factor influencing tick populations and disease transmission. The availability of host species like deer and rodents, human behavior and activities, and other ecosystem disturbances also play significant roles. Addressing the complex interactions between climate, land use, and tick-borne disease dynamics is crucial for developing effective prevention and control strategies.

This chapter addresses the connections between climate change and KFD, which is essential for developing effective strategies to prevent and control this emerging public health threat in India.

Ticks: Tiny Terrors with a Big Bite and the Spread of Disease

Ticks are a unique category of ectoparasites that feed exclusively on blood, known to people worldwide. They transmit a wider variety of disease-causing pathogens than any other group of arthropods, including viral, bacterial, protozoan, and even fungal agents. Additionally, ticks cause annoying or even fatal injuries to animals and humans due to immobilization, toxins, or severe allergic reactions to their bites.

Body Structure

The anterior capitulum, which houses the mouthparts, and the idiosoma, which has eight walking legs, are the two primary areas that make up the tick body.

Ticks are apex predators without a head and a strongly united body without a distinct abdomen and thorax. The chelicerae, which are small, paired appendages that pierce the skin, the food canal for blood intake, and the paired segmented palps, which give sensory data for identification of the host, are all parts of the capitulum. The hypostome [toothed] is what embeds the tick into the skin of the host. In Argasid ticks, capitulum is recessed behind the front extension of the body [7].

On the ventral surface of the rest of the body are the spiracles, genital pores, and anus. Hard ticks, commonly known as ixodid ticks, have a noticeable scutum on their dorsal surface resembling a plate. In contrast to ixodid ticks, Argasid ticks, also referred to as soft ticks, have a velvety outer cuticle with no scutum [8].

The hemocoel, a straightforward open cavity that houses the internal organs, is filled with hemolymph, circulating throughout the tick body. Ticks lack hemoglobin, just as other terrestrial arthropods, and the hemolymph is ineffective in carrying oxygen. The largest internal organ, the midgut, comprises multiple lateral diverticula and a central sac-like stomach that occupies most of the interior space of the animal [9]. The reproductive organs and the paired salivary glands, which resemble white grape-like clusters, are two more notable internal organs. The reproductive system of female ticks consists of the seminal receptacle, uterus, paired oviducts, ovary, and vagina, which links to the genital pore. The ovary grows and swells up with huge, brown, or amber-colored eggs during feeding. The seminal vesicle, testis, vasa deferentia, and ejaculatory duct, which join the genital pore, make up the reproductive system of male ticks. Most of this is obscured by a large, multilobed white accessory gland, which produces components of the sac-like spermatophore used by the male tick to transfer sperm to the female. The respiratory system is composed of many tracheal tubes that are connected to the marginal spiracles. In contrast, the excretory sac and Malpighian tubules, which are linked to the anal hole, are responsible for eliminating waste. The two coxal glands of argasid ticks expel extra water and salts gathered while eating through the coxal pores. The body's synganglion, or united central nervous system, is above the genital pore [8, 9].

Systematic Classification and Relationships

Phylum: Arthropoda
Subphylum: Mandibulata
Class: Arachnida
Subclass: Acari
Super Order: Parasitiformes
Order: Ixodida

Family: *Ixodidae Anocentor, Amblyomma, Dermacentor, Boophilus, Haemaphysalis, Hyalomma Rhipicephalus, Ixodes* *Argasidae Argas, Otobius, Ornithodorus,* *Nuttalliellidae Nuttalliella*

Ticks belong to the Arachnida class, which also includes scorpions and spiders. Arachnids lack mandibles and instead have chelicerae, which are scissor- or pincer-like appendages used for cutting. They are without antennae and lack a definite head or thorax. Ticks and mites are members of the Acari subclass. They are a part of the acarine order Parasitiformes' Ixodida suborder. Three families comprise the Ixodida suborder: Ixodidae, Argasidae, and Nuttalliellidae. With over 650 species, the Ixodidae family, also known as hard ticks, is the largest [10].

Ixodid ticks are essential disease carriers that impact both livestock and wildlife. They undergo three active life stages, including a single nymphal stage. The genus Ixodes, which is representative of Prostriata and has an anterior anal groove, and the 13 genera that makeup Metastriata, which have a posterior anal groove, are the other divisions of the Ixodidae family [9, 11].

Argasidae

The soft-bodied ticks in the Argasidae family have a leathery, highly adaptable cuticle. Approximately 170 species are grouped into five genera. Often, ticks undergo three active life stages, but most species possess many nymphal stages prior to maturing into adults. The approximately 100 species of ticks in the genus Ornithodoros have a rounded body edge and a velvety cuticle with numerous tiny bumps, known as mammillae. Most soft ticks do not play a substantial role in disease transmission, except those carrying the recurrent fever-causing spirochetes [12].

Nuttalliellidae

The third tick family, Nuttalliellidae, is represented by a single species, *Nuttalliella namaqua*, found in Southern Africa. Nuttalliellidae is monospecific. This family possesses traits shared by the other two tick families. Its scutum of ixodid ticks resembles the dorsal pseudoscutum, and its cuticle, characterized by creases, crevices, and heights, resembles argasid ticks.

During the Mesozoic era, when the dinosaurs lived, ticks were already a highly evolved and ancient group of Acarines. After being found in New Jersey amber, a larval tick was dated to the upper Cretaceous period, with an estimated age of 90–94 million years [12].

Decoding the Tick Biology: Life Cycle of the Tick

Ticks undergo four main stages: egg, larval, nymph, and adult. All of them, except maybe the egg, need to feed on blood to grow. Most tick species require three different hosts, one for each stage. After feeding, they detach and progress to the next stage. Adult females, after a big blood meal, lay eggs and then die. Ticks can wait long between meals, stretching their life cycle for years, especially for some argasid ticks. The leading tick families, Ixodidae and Argasidae, have critical differences in their life cycles [13].

Life Cycles of Ixodid Ticks

Ixodid ticks have slow feeding cycles lasting from a few days to two weeks. Ticks feed on the blood of immature and adult hosts, except for certain species' non-feeding males. When these ticks locate a host, they use their mouthparts to pierce the host's skin, and then their salivary glands release a cement-like substance around the wound to hold them in place. The ticks are securely anchored by the cement, making it extremely difficult to remove them. Ticks release potent anticoagulants and anti-inflammatory chemicals while feeding, which impede the healing of the host's wound and stimulate blood flow. To handle their huge blood diets, which can increase their body weight by 10 to 100 times, ticks create new cuticles while they feed.

Tick females only eat once. Although it can occur before attachment, mating in the genus *Ixodes* typically takes place while the ticks are feeding on a host. In metastriate Ixodidae (ixodid ticks excluding the genus *Ixodes*), mating occurs within a few days after the start of feeding. Mating is triggered by sex pheromones, which include volatile 2,6-dichlorophenol and nonvolatile cholesteryl esters that are present on the tick's surface of the body.

Within 24 to 48 hours of mating, female ticks devour large amounts of blood and expand dramatically. When entirely gorged, they leave their hosts and look for a safe place to lay hundreds of eggs. For example, *Dermacentor variabilis*, the American dog tick, typically lays over 5,000 eggs.

The female tick perishes after producing eggs. Male ticks can mate several times, feeding between each mating; however, they only expand a little during feeding, in contrast to female ticks. Mating can occur on or off the host in certain Ixodes species, including the sheep tick [*Ixodes ricinus*] and the tick with black legs [*Ixodes scapularis*]. Males of some Ixodes species that live in nests always mate off of their hosts and have vestiges of their hypostomes. Thousands of larvae hatch from their eggs and start looking for hosts.

In contrast to species that live in nests, these larvae spread into the foliage and come into contact with animals that pass by. As previously mentioned, the larvae dig into the skin after connecting to a host, form a feeding pool, and feed. Usually, this feeding procedure takes two to four days. The larvae separate from the host once they are engorged and molt on the ground. Typically, a microhabitat that is sheltered, such as soil, leaf litter, or the nests of the hosts, is the site of molting. Nymphal stage and adult ticks must locate a new host and food source after molting. Nonetheless, they live off the host for over 90% of their life cycle. Ticks that search for hosts and feed during each of the three parasitic stages are said to have a three-host life cycle.

Certain Ixodid species have either a single-host or two-host life cycle. For example, the cattle tick *Boophilus annulatus* has a one-host life cycle in which all stages of feeding, molting, and even breeding occur on the same host, whereas the camel tick *Hyalomma dromedarii* consists of a life cycle between two hosts, on which the larvae and nymphs feed [13].

Life Cycles of Argasid Ticks

Argasid ticks, also known as soft ticks, are known for their rapid feeding habits. They embed their mouthparts, like ixodid ticks, after crawling onto a host, but they do not form a cement-like substance. Bloodsucking happens quickly, and while the ticks continue to feed, they secrete copious volumes of a colorless, transparent fluid called coxal fluid. This fluid may occasionally be discharged shortly after feeding begins. Ticks may concentrate on how they feed and regulate their water balance internally by employing the coxal fluid to eliminate excess water and salts.

Depending on how flexible their cuticle is, ticks can swell to a weight of five to ten times their initial mass after feeding. After feeding, which takes as little as 30 to 60 minutes, mature ticks depart to undergo molting or lay eggs in the case of females. Multiple gonotrophic cycles are the mechanism by which female Argasid ticks deposit little quantities of eggs [typically 500 eggs per batch] following every session of feeding. The time taken between those feedings is usually a few months, but it can be as long as many years if hosts are unavailable. Usually, mating takes place far from the host. Argasid ticks have a long lifespan because they undergo several nymphal stages, ranging from six to seven in certain species. They also exhibit a strong resilience to famine, which increases their lifespan. As such, the entire life cycle of these ticks can take ten to twenty years.

Most Argasid tick larvae look for hosts after laying eggs and hatching, eat quickly, and molt into the nymphal stage first. Those nymphs then molt into the second nymphal stage, search for hosts once more, and feed quickly. After that, the life cycle exhibits a great deal of variety, sometimes entailing further nymphal phases before adulthood and, in other instances, proceeding straight to the adult stage. Males often go through fewer nymphal stages and emerge earlier than females. Some Argasid species, especially those that parasitize bats, have larvae that remain attached to their hosts for a prolonged period, feeding at a snail's pace similar to that of ixodid ticks, and then undergo two molts without feeding again.

Following this phase, the life cycle of the majority of Argasid ticks resumes its typical pattern. *Otobius megnini* is another unusual species that only has one nymphal stage. Known as autogeny, females produce eggs without requiring a blood meal, and neither sex requires a blood meal.

Beyond Bloodsuckers: The Hidden Lives of Ticks

As hematophagous ectoparasites, ticks seek out particular environmental conditions to carry out their life cycle, which includes the stages of egg-laying, larval development, nymphal development, and adulthood. For them to actively search for hosts, temperatures over 7°C and high humidity levels [>85%] are necessary. Ticks consume blood from competent hosts, such as humans, or from incompetent hosts, like other animals, once they have located a suitable host. Ticks play a crucial role in disease transmission because they can transmit them to hosts while feeding, without necessarily resulting in death, which can impact host health.

They navigate their existence intricately linked to environmental factors, such as host availability, weather conditions, and climate. These elements play pivotal roles in shaping natural foci, specialized habitats where ticks flourish. The interplay of temperature, humidity, and the presence of hosts within the larger ecosystem and specific microclimates further determines their distribution and abundance.

At the forefront of tick survival strategies is Haller's organ, a sophisticated sensory apparatus located on their first pair of legs. This organ enables ticks to sense their surroundings comprehensively, detecting vital cues like body heat, odor, shadows, and movement-induced vibrations. These sensory inputs are crucial for ticks to identify and locate potential hosts necessary for their life cycle progression.

Despite spending most of their lives away from vertebrate hosts, hard ticks must secure blood meals to advance through their developmental stages. This necessity underscores their adaptive strategies, utilizing a combination of sensory and behavioral mechanisms to meet their physiological needs. For instance, ticks employ efficient strategies to absorb humidity and minimize water loss, with species like *Ixodes ricinus* relying exclusively on air moisture absorption rather than drinking water. They also adjust their activity patterns to specific times of day and seek out shelters with optimal microclimate conditions, guided by sensitive thermoreceptor cells.

Ticks further enhance their survival through chemosensors located on their mouthparts and legs, which detect chemical signals from potential hosts. This sensory capability enables ticks to locate and feed on suitable hosts, which is essential for acquiring blood meals necessary for growth and reproduction. The duration of these blood meals varies significantly across different life stages of ticks; for instance, in *Ixodes ricinus*, larvae may feed for just two days, whereas adult females can extend their feeding period up to ten days.

During feeding, ticks undergo physiological processes that concentrate the ingested blood, making it three to five times denser, while excess water is expelled back into the host through a pump mechanism. This activity is crucial for transmitting pathogens from ticks to hosts *via* their salivary glands, highlighting the role of ticks as vectors for various infectious diseases.

Female ticks, in particular, undergo remarkable physiological changes during a blood meal, potentially increasing their body mass by up to 200 times. To manage this tremendous influx of blood, ticks require intricate structural and anatomical adjustments to prevent bursting. The gut epithelium and cuticle expand in the initial days after feeding, optimizing blood absorption efficiency. Notably, morphological changes in ticks only commence in the final 12 to 24 hours of the feeding process, marking a critical stage in their physiological adaptation to the blood meal cycle.

In summary, ticks' ability to thrive hinges on their ability to sense environmental cues, secure blood meals, and navigate complex physiological adaptations during feeding. Comprehending these mechanisms is crucial for understanding the dynamics of tick-borne illness transmission and highlights the complex interrelationship among ticks, their hosts, and their environment.

Tick Ecology, Seasonal Triggers and Host Seeking Behaviour

Most ticks are exophilic, meaning they are not nidicolous and can be found freely in various habitats, including grassy meadows, brushlands, savannahs, woods, and even sandy semidesert regions. These exophilic ticks live outside their host's body and are not active year-round. They have specific seasons when the weather is just right for them to grow and reproduce. When they are searching for a host, this active period is referred to as host-seeking behavior. They enter a low-power mode called diapause for the remainder of the year [14].

On the other hand, some ticks are nidicolous, meaning they prefer to live in the cracks, crevices, caves, and buildings where their hosts take refuge. Many species of Ixodes ticks and most Argasid ticks have this behavior. Argasid ticks often live near their hosts in cozy nests or burrows and do not follow the usual seasonal activity pattern. However, some Argasid ticks have figured out a clever way to hitch a ride. Species coexisting with migrating birds or bats will wait for the host's appearance to correspond with the host's return to the nest.

In cooler areas, such as temperate and subantarctic regions, tick behavior follows a remarkably precise seasonal rhythm. Three things set the tick active:

Warmer weather: As the temperature rises, ticks wake up ready for action.

Daylight hours: Longer days signal it is time to search for a host.

Sunshine: Solar energy helps fuel their activity.

Ambush or Hunter? Tick Strategies for Finding a Host

Once active, ticks have two main strategies for finding a host:

Ambush

These ticks climb vegetation, with adults reaching the highest points, and wait patiently for a passing animal to brush against them. Like a tiny hitchhiker, they latch on for a blood meal.

Hunter

Some tick species act more like hunters in drier areas with less cover. They emerge from their hiding spots and actively move towards animals, following their scent [or, rarely, sound] for a delicious meal.

Ecological Impacts on Tick Biology and Pathogen Transmission Dynamics

Tick ecology is closely related to how they interact with biotic and abiotic elements of their surroundings, fundamentally influencing the temporal and spatial variation in the tick-borne pathogen infections. As blood-sucking parasites, ticks' biological environment comprises their hosts, which react to their presence over short and long terms, exerting physiological and evolutionary pressures on ticks. Despite being intermittent parasites, spending much of their off-host life cycle, ticks are subject to environmental phenomena, such as the structure of the habitat and climate, which significantly impact their development and survival.

Ixodid ticks, characterized by taking one [or a few in the case of some Argasid ticks] huge blood meal per life stage, undergo inter-stadial periods off-host. These periods can last from weeks to months or even years, depending on the temperature, during which ticks molt to the next life cycle stage. Exceptions like *Boophilus microplus* and *Hyalomma anatolicum excavatum*, known as two- and one-host ticks, respectively, remain on the host through one or more interstadial periods.

At an individual level, ticks' potential as vectors is enhanced by their strategy of taking large, prolonged blood meals and their adaptations to evade the host's defenses. However, at a population level, their potential vector aspect is limited by the necessity of consuming fewer meals per stage. The rate of contact between vectors and hosts is constrained, with one host species limited to just one contact per generation. Moreover, ticks must acquire pathogens during a blood meal and molt to the following stage before being able to pass the infection stage to another host, a process critical for their role as vectors. Maintaining infection across stages [including transovarial transmission from female to larvae] is essential for sustained transmission cycles.

Climate-driven seasonal population dynamics have a significant influence on the transmission dynamics of ticks and their associated pathogens. Variations in temperature and other climatic factors affect tick activity, development rates, and survival, influencing pathogen transmission's pace and intensity. Longer delays in transmission due to seasonal or geographic climate variations can slow down transmission cycles, while tick mortality rates also fluctuate in response to climatic conditions.

Population dynamics further dictate the seasonal variations of ticks that are active and ready to quest for hosts, directly impacting the infection risk. Understanding these ecological and biological intricacies is crucial for predicting and managing the spread of tick-borne diseases, as shifts in climate patterns continue to alter the dynamics of tick populations and their interactions with hosts.

Ticks and Climate Change: Understanding the Relationship

It is predicted that environmental changes, including climate change, will heighten the risk for Tick-Borne Diseases [TBDs] and tick-borne illnesses in several ways. Among these are expected increases in the count, spread, and behavior of different tick species, as well as the diseases they carry. It is anticipated that shifting weather patterns may increase the habitats of animal reservoirs and hosts, increasing the interactions between ticks, hosts, and people across longer seasons. Furthermore, when temperatures change, human activities are likely to adjust, which could lead to an extension in the duration of human-tick habitat contact. A variety of environmental factors shape tick and host ecosystems, in addition to those caused by changes in climate.

Rising temperatures are known to broaden the spread and increase the abundance and activity of rodents and deer, impacting the dynamics of populations of ticks and the transmission of Tick-Borne Diseases [TBDs]. Reservoir hosts, such as wild rodents, particularly mice, are crucial for providing pathogens to immature tick stages in the transmission cycle of TBDs. Meanwhile, reproduction hosts, primarily deer, supply blood meals necessary for adult female ticks to reproduce [14].

There is a distinct seasonal activity pattern for ticks based on stage. After the first monsoon rains in June, adults start to move around. Their population peaks in July and August, then gradually declines in September. Female ticks lay a large number of eggs, which hatch into larvae after feeding. Under the forest litter, these larvae are latent and only begin to grow during the monsoon season. They come out to play during the post-monsoon season, which is usually from October to December, when the litter dries up. January through May is the peak period for nymphal activity, which is strongly linked to epidemics. Nymphs are therefore considered the most important stage in human transmission. Although bigger animals like cattle and monkeys are excellent hosts for tick reproduction, adult ticks only have a minor role in tick reproduction (Fig. **2**).

Climatic and Environmental Factors Shaping Tick Dynamics

Tick species each have preferred biomes and environmental conditions that dictate their geographic distribution and the associated risk areas for humans. Microhabitat factors like soil characteristics play a crucial role in tick survival and the establishment of new populations. Changes in habitat features due to climate change, such as fragmentation, biodiversity loss, resource availability, and land use, profoundly impact tick dynamics, animal hosts, and human exposure to ticks. For instance, Lyme Disease [LD] emerged in the United States during the 1970s due to reforestation leading to increased deer populations, facilitating the expansion of *Ixodes scapularis* ticks carrying *B. burgdorferi*. This historical example illustrates how ecological changes can influence tick-borne disease dynamics by altering host availability and habitat suitability [15].

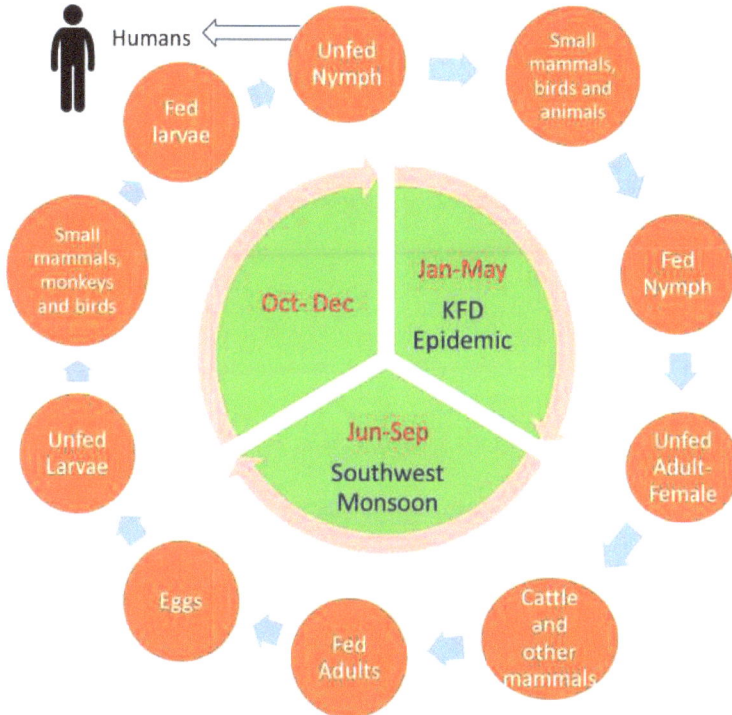

Fig. (2). Kyasanur Forest Disease [KFD]: A life disease.

The tick *Dermacentor variabilis* exhibits excellent adaptability, varying according to location and climate. It has a one-year life cycle in warmer southern regions, with larvae emerging in spring and adults active in early summer. In the cooler north, colder soil and shorter days delay larval emergence and development, forcing the tick to take two years to complete its life cycle. This life cycle variation allows *D. variabilis* to thrive in various habitats across its territory.

Unlike *Dermacentor variabilis*, the *Ixodes scapularis* tick has a unique life cycle strategy. While both have nymphs and larvae that fccd during the summer and spring seasons, *Ixodes scapularis* [the mature ones] become active in early spring and fall, with the larval and nymphal feeding stages reversed. Infected nymphs feed on mice in spring and summer, creating a reservoir of infected animals. Then, in the fall, these adult ticks feed on other mammals, potentially including humans, transmitting the disease.

The variations in tick life cycle, like the one seen in *Ixodes scapularis*, significantly impact how diseases spread in wildlife and human populations. Understanding these life cycles is crucial for controlling the spread of tick-borne diseases.

Typically, tick population dynamics are primarily dependent on temperature-dependent development rates, closely related to tick adaptability to their natural habitat. The rapid laying of enormous egg masses by female Ixodid ticks makes the rate of development between stages a crucial demographic element. Tick development rates increase nonlinearly with rising ambient temperature, just like those of other poikilothermic species. Determining these temperature-dependent rates in carefully regulated laboratory environments is crucial for precisely projecting growth timelines in various geographical locations. Field measurements may be sufficient in equatorial locations with consistent temperatures, whereas laboratory investigations yield more accurate data in regions with seasonal changes. Ticks optimize their life cycles in response to environmental cues, which affects their population dynamics and distribution patterns, as demonstrated by this physiological adaptation [15].

Tick Responses to Climate Envelopes: Adaptations and Implications

Like all living things, ticks function inside certain climate envelopes that determine the climatic conditions necessary for their dispersal and survival. Due to their limited climatic ranges, several tick species are highly vulnerable to temperature alterations, which can significantly affect their population densities and geographical distributions. On the other hand, species with broad climatic tolerances, such as *Ixodes ricinus*, can survive throughout large geographical regions. For example, *I. ricinus* is a flexible generalist tick that can be found throughout Europe, from the Caspian Sea to the Atlantic coast, from Arctic Norway to North Africa, and even at elevations of up to 1,500 meters in the European Alps.

Similar to this, *Ixodes scapularis* is a generalist feeder that inhabits almost the whole eastern United States as well as parts of Canada. Climate change is expected to have the greatest impact on the outer boundaries of the latitudinal and altitudinal ranges of these widely distributed species. For example, ticks, such as *I. scapularis* and *I. ricinus*, may be adaptively resilient to present climatic changes, despite possible alterations to local seasons and host communities. Their capacity to use a variety of hosts, such as reindeer and white-tailed and red deer, may allow them to alter their ranges instead of suffering from severe contractions.

Changes in host populations can indirectly impact tick distribution and abundance due to climate change. Since they may feed on various land animals, generalist ticks like *Ixodes ricinus* and *Ixodes scapularis* are unlikely to be significantly harmed by these changes. The effects of climate change on the populations of ticks that are more specific to their hosts, such as the bat tick *Ixodes vespertilionis*, which are long-legged, could significantly impact the ticks themselves [16].

Although rare, data sets from the same places are necessary to show how climate change affects tick populations and the risk and incidence of tick-borne diseases. A link between changes in tick populations or illness incidence and a changing climate does not necessarily prove causation, even in cases where such data sets are available. Climate change is the cause, if more data confirm this correlation and show responses to particular climate factors while excluding changes that are consistent with other putative drivers of host populations. Tick-borne diseases, hosts, habitat, climate, and tick models can all be used to suggest possible drivers.

Moreover, it is difficult to separate the mechanisms underlying variations in tick abundance and dispersion, as well as tick-borne illnesses. It is challenging to determine whether these changes are directly caused by climate change or indirectly by alterations in hosts, habitat, or human behavior resulting from climate change, all of which increase the risk of exposure. Furthermore, climate conditions rarely affect hosts, environments, or human behavior. This makes it even more challenging to determine whether changes in diseases carried by ticks are ultimately caused by climate change or other variables that affect host populations, such as anthropogenic land use or wildlife management.

Overall, the extensive range and great ecological adaptability of generalist ticks imply that they could adapt to and benefit from climate change by adjusting their host choices and geographic ranges. Their adaptability highlights their ecological flexibility and resilience in the face of changing environmental conditions [16].

Mechanisms Driving the Impact of Climate Change on Ticks and Tick-Borne Diseases

According to recent trends of climate change, the world's temperature has risen by an average of 1°C during the period of preindustry [1850–1900], and it was estimated that by 2081–2100, temperatures would increase by 1.5–2°C. However, the world is not warming at the same rate. For example, land temperatures are rising faster than ocean temperatures, and the Arctic is predicted to witness far more significant temperature increases than most other locations. Not only is the temperature fluctuating, but the patterns of rainfall are also changing. While some countries, particularly those in arid regions, are dealing with more prolonged and frequent droughts, specific locations are experiencing a rise in rainfall and an increase in extreme weather events, such as stronger winds, larger rainstorms, and more frequent flooding.

Since ticks primarily feed on their hosts, abiotic environmental changes significantly impact them, and many factors related to climate change are also expected to have an impact. For instance, research on *I. ricinus* has demonstrated that increased temperatures hasten the rates of oviposition, egg development, and interstadial development. Studies have demonstrated that a higher percentage of the *I. ricinus* population becomes active at higher temperatures. Numerous studies have also demonstrated that *I. ricinus* activity is impacted by saturation deficit, which is the capacity of air to dry that is influenced by both relative humidity and temperature [17].

Thus, chilly temperatures that slow life cycle progression and activity likely define the cooler limits of the climatic envelope for ticks with environmental requirements similar to those of *Ixodes ricinus*. Since *I. ricinus* finds it difficult to live for long at temperatures below -15°C, these borders may also be defined by more significant winter mortality at higher elevations and latitudes. *I. ricinus* benefits from greater life cycle rates and activity further south, where temperatures are warm; nevertheless, temperatures over 30°C, even with high humidity [above 80%], result in much higher mortality, which may indicate the southern limits of their distribution. Higher tick densities raise the chances of more ticks biting [and so acquiring infection from] a host when it is infectious, which is relevant to the rates of disease transmission [18].

Apart from the factors that determine the development of ticks, including oviposition, fertility, activity, and mortality, changes in climate can also impact the seasonal phenology of several stages of ticks, such as larvae, nymphs, and adults. More larvae will contract the infection if the peak of nymphs and larvae occurs simultaneously each season. Therefore, the possibility of disease transmission may alter if climate change causes a shift in the seasonal maxima of certain tick stages.

Tick populations and disease prevalence can be impacted by environment and host abundance, which can have a domino effect on tick populations even in situations where a change in climate does not directly impact tick demography. It is not always difficult to demonstrate a bridge between changes in host abundance, land usage, or ecology and the occurrence of tick-borne illnesses, assuming the data are available. It can be challenging to determine whether climate change is the primary cause of these indirect impacts and to weigh its influence against other possible causes.

Although climate change can affect ticks' habitats and abundance, knowing the exact number of ticks is more advantageous for researchers when assessing the risk of tick bites, as it is harder to measure accurately. Most common methods for detecting ticks, such as counting them on animals or dragging clothes through grass, only find ticks that are actively looking for a meal. This activity can vary significantly depending on the season and weather conditions. Due to this, even though the ideal way to measure climate change's impact would be to count all the ticks, many studies rely on simply finding out if ticks are present in an area. This approach might not be as sensitive to change, and some details may be missed, but it is easier to measure accurately and compare across different studies.

For people, the most critical measure is how many people get sick in a specific area, like the number of cases per 10,000 people. For tick researchers, a key measure is how many infected ticks [especially young ticks called nymphs] are in the environment. This can be a good indicator of human risk.

Another measure, the percentage of ticks carrying a specific disease, is less helpful for understanding how likely people are to get bitten by an infected tick. However, it remains interesting for scientists because it helps them understand how different animals play a key role in disease spread.

These different measures could be affected by climate change in various ways. Some only depend on how long ticks live and how active they are. Others are also influenced by the types and numbers of animals available for ticks to feed on. Finally, the number of people getting sick is also influenced by the population density in a particular area and the behavior of its residents. Due to this, it is essential to pay attention to which measure is used when examining studies on tick-borne diseases and climate change.

The aforementioned challenges in distinguishing the effects of climate change from those of hosts, habitat, or human activities, as well as the measurement errors in various adjoining parameters like disease incidence, presence of a tick, pathogen prevalence, tick abundance, or risk, must be considered when concluding climate change's impact on tick-borne diseases [19].

Evidence of Climate Change Effects on Ticks

Our planet's warming climate is causing a ripple effect across ecosystems, and one tiny creature taking advantage is the *Ixodes ricinus*. This tick, known for transmitting Lyme disease, is undergoing a significant range shift, expanding its boundaries further north and at higher altitudes. For *I. ricinus*, areas with specific temperature ranges are used to limit its spread. These areas act as a kind of "no entry zone" at the edges of its usual habitat. However, climate change alters these temperature zones, allowing ticks to thrive in previously unsuitable locations.

The evidence for this range shift is compelling. In Europe, *I. ricinus* has begun a northward migration. In Arctic Norway, the tick's range has advanced to an impressive 69°N latitude—approximately 400 kilometers farther north than in the 1940s. Similarly, Sweden has witnessed the tick climb from below 61°N to a much higher 66°N since the 1980s. *I. ricinus* is not just expanding horizontally; it is also scaling new heights. In the Czech Republic, the tick's upper altitude limit has increased from around 700 meters in the 1950s to a significantly higher 1,100 meters in the 2000s. This upward shift suggests that even mountain regions are becoming hospitable for these bloodsuckers [20].

The case of the UK is still more interesting. Here, the increase in *I. ricinus* population might not be directly linked to climate change. Instead, this could be the rising deer population, which serves as a primary breeding ground for these ticks. Milder winters, likely brought on by climate change, create ideal conditions for deer to thrive, indirectly leading to a higher tick population.

Researchers are using sophisticated models to predict the future of *I. ricinus* under a changing climate. In Scotland, one such model suggests that warming temperatures will extend the tick's active season and allow it to occupy higher altitudes. This, in turn, could significantly increase the risk of tick-borne diseases. Additionally, ecological niche modeling across Europe forecasts a northward and eastward expansion of *I. ricinus*, further highlighting the potential threat.

Thus, climate change is undoubtedly playing a pivotal role in the range shift. This shift has a two-fold impact: it expands the tick's geographical reach and increases the risk of tick-borne diseases, such as KFD. The interplay between climate, host populations such as deer, and tick activity highlights the intricate web of ecological changes occurring in the world.

Canada's natural landscapes are renowned for their beauty and diversity, but climate change is also influencing the tick population. Tick species, such as *Ixodes scapularis* and *Amblyomma americanum*, are expected to experience significant changes in distribution and abundance due to a warming planet. Scientists have used detailed models to predict the future of *Ixodes scapularis*, a tick known for transmitting Lyme disease. These models suggest that as temperatures rise, tick populations will survive better and expand beyond their current range. This "climate envelope" refers to a species' specific temperature conditions for thriving. With warmer weather, this envelope expands northward, potentially allowing the tick to invade cooler regions of Canada.

The *Amblyomma americanum* [lone star tick] is already causing problems in the southeastern United States, spreading diseases like Ehrlichia and tularemia. Historical records revealed a gradual northward expansion toward the Canadian border dating back to the 1890s. While the exact reasons for this development are not immediately apparent, models based on temperature suitability align with these observed patterns. These models forecast that the change in climate will further accelerate this northward expansion, enabling the lone star tick to establish populations in previously unsuitable, colder regions of Canada [21].

In Brazil, the *Amblyomma cajennense* tick complex, known for transmitting spotted fever, might experience a range contraction due to climate change. Models predict that future climate scenarios will make the environment less suitable for these ticks, potentially decreasing their prevalence and positively impacting public health by reducing spotted fever cases.

On the other hand, climate change in Argentina and Australia is not only causing warming; it is also changing rainfall patterns. This creates a fascinating contrast in how it affects the cattle tick, *Boophilus microplus*. In areas expected to receive more rain, models suggest an expansion of *B. microplus* populations. This is terrible news for the beef cattle industry, as increased tick populations lead to more infestations, reduced livestock productivity, and animal health issues.

While some tick species are expanding their territories with rising temperatures, others might face a shrinking habitat. This regional variation highlights the complexity of the issue and the need for location-specific approaches.

Different tick species have unique needs and adaptations; some thrive in this new environment, while others struggle. Ticks like *Ixodes ricinus* and *Ixodes scapularis* prefer relaxed, moist environments. They are susceptible to how quickly moisture evaporates, a factor called saturation deficit. Unfortunately for them, climate change is bringing warmer temperatures that also tend to decrease saturation deficit. This creates a northward expansion opportunity for these tick species, allowing them to move into previously unsuitable territories.

On the other hand, some tick species, like *Ornithodoros sonrai* and *Ornithodoros marocanus*, prefer hot and dry climates. These desert-dwellers have been observed increasing in abundance and expanding their range in places like Northwest Morocco and Senegal. Frequently droughts, a hallmark of climate change in these regions and their drier conditions, are likely to create ideal habitats for these heat-loving ticks, allowing them to multiply and spread further. These contrasting responses highlight the complex interplay between climate change and tick biology. Some species benefit from the new normal, expanding their range and potentially increasing the risk of tick-borne diseases they carry. However, others might find their preferred habitats shrinking or face ecological disruptions limiting their populations.

These contrasting examples showcase the intricate relationship between climate and ticks. Not only are temperatures rising, but other environmental elements like rainfall patterns are also essential. Some tick species might thrive under new conditions, expanding their range and potentially increasing the spread of diseases. However, others might find their habitat shrinking or facing ecological changes that reduce disease risks. This highlights the importance of considering variables beyond temperature when assessing the impact of climate change on tick populations. Precipitation patterns and other environmental variables must also be taken into account.

Nuanced Strategies to Consider

Species-specific Needs

Different tick species have different ecological requirements. Understanding these needs helps us predict how they will respond to climate change.

Climate Variables

Temperature is just one criterion. Rainfall patterns, humidity, and other factors also play a role.

Regional Variations

Climate change does not affect all places equally. Considering regional environmental changes enables us to develop targeted mitigation strategies.

By integrating these factors, researchers can better anticipate and manage the impacts of climate change on tick populations and public health risks they pose. This way, we can protect ourselves and our ecosystems from the tick-borne threats of a changing climate.

In conclusion, the world of ticks is complex, with diverse species exhibiting a range of adaptations to survive and thrive in various climates. These adaptations, particularly those influencing life cycle timing and host-seeking behavior, are crucial in transmitting tick-borne diseases. Thus, understanding these intricate tick-borne disease cycles is paramount for developing effective prevention and control strategies.

This understanding becomes especially critical when examining Kyasanur Forest Disease [KFD], a viral tick-borne hemorrhagic fever posing a significant public health threat. Thus, the other half of this chapter delves deeper into the world of KFD, exploring its epidemiology, clinical presentation, and the challenges associated with its control.

Kyasanur Forest Disease [KFD]: An Introduction

The Kyasanur Forest Disease [KFD] is a zoonotic illness that causes a sudden, high fever along with other symptoms like diarrhea, prostration, nausea, and sometimes even hemorrhagic and neurological symptoms. Humans contract KFD through tick bites, and the virus that causes KFD belongs to the Flavivirus genus within the Flaviviridae family. First discovered in 1957 in the forested area of Kyasanur in Shimoga district, Karnataka state, the virus was named after the dense forest where it was initially identified. It is also known as "monkey disease" or "monkey fever" because it is associated with fatalities among monkeys in affected areas. However, it remains unclear why it emerged in the mid-1950s. Through serological and genomic characterization, a variation of the Kyasanur Forest Disease Virus [KFDV] was identified as the Alkhurma Hemorrhagic Fever Virus [AHFV], recently discovered in Saudi Arabia. The 89% sequence homology between KFDV and AHFV suggests they most likely have the exact evolutionary origin. Some researchers suggest that the divergence of these viruses occurred approximately seven hundred years ago.

Numerous creatures, including rats, mice, shrews, squirrels, porcupines, and hares, are thought to act as reservoir hosts for the disease. Nymphs, a stage in the life cycle of the forest tick *Haemaphysalis spinigera*, serve as a vehicle *via* which human disease can be spread through biting. Within the genus *Flavivirus* and family Flaviviridae, KFDV belongs to the category of mammalian tick-borne viruses, formerly called the tick-borne encephalitis serogroup.

A Legacy of Monkey Fever: A Historical Perspective

Monkeys and humans are incidental hosts, with wild monkeys highly susceptible and amplifying outbreaks. No clinical disease has been observed in other wild or domestic animals. Symptoms of KFD include sudden fever, muscle pain, headache, swollen lymph nodes, and pain in the upper chest and neck. Hemorrhages mainly involve gastrointestinal bleeding and bleeding from the gums and nose. In some cases, during recovery, encephalitis may manifest as tremors, neck stiffness, mental disturbances, and muscle weakness.

In India, the case fatality rate of Kyasanur Forest Disease (KFD) ranges from 3% to 10%. Experimental infections in langurs and bonnet monkeys demonstrated high levels of viremia and mortality rates of up to 85%. Infected monkeys showed lymphopenia, anemia, elevated liver enzymes, and diarrhea, with significant lymphoid lesions in lymph nodes, spleen, and intestines but no hemorrhages. Monkeys thus serve as a good model for studying KFD. The virus also causes lethal disease in juvenile BALB/c mice without adaptation, with animals dying within 4–5 days. Despite these findings, the disease's mechanisms are poorly understood, highlighting the need for an animal model. In 1995, a similar virus, Alkhumra Virus [ALKV], was identified in patients with hemorrhagic fever and central nervous system symptoms in Saudi Arabia. ALKV has a 25% mortality rate, primarily affecting sheep handlers, butchers, and meat consumers. Given the genetic similarity between ALKV and KFDV, KFD models may aid in the study of ALKV.

Following its discovery, KFD was mainly reported in Shimoga, Uttara Kannada, Udupi, Dakshina Kannada, and Chikkamagaluru districts in Karnataka for over 50 years. In November 2012, KFD was detected outside its endemic zone in the National Park at Bandipur, Karnataka, with subsequent cases in Maddur Forest Range, Chamarajanagar, and Wayanad, Kerala. Between 2013 and 2015, KFD was reported in humans and monkeys in Wayanad and among tribals in Mallapuram, Kerala. Occupational exposure was noted among cashew nut workers in Goa, with ongoing KFD activity since 2015. In 2016, an outbreak in Dodamarg taluka, Sindhudurg district, Maharashtra, resulted in 130 reported cases.

Although initially restricted to five districts in Karnataka, KFD has spread along the Western Ghats in five states. Antibodies to KFDV were detected in other parts of India, including West Bengal, Rajasthan, Gujarat, and the Andaman and Nicobar Islands, suggesting potential undetected KFDV activity beyond known outbreak areas. The KFD virus was initially suspected of belonging to the Russian Spring-Summer [RSS] complex of viruses. Currently, KFD is reported only from India. However, some closely related viruses to KFD include:

- The Omsk hemorrhagic fever virus -Siberia.
- The Nanjianyin virus - China.
- The Alkhurma virus - Saudi Arabia [22].

Understanding KFD Through the Lens of Epidemiology

Kyasanur Forest Disease [KFD] is not a random occurrence. Its emergence, persistence, and spread can be explained through the lens of epidemiology, a field related to illness in populations, including its patterns, effects, and consequences. A key concept in epidemiology is the epidemiological triad, which considers three crucial factors that influence the outbreak and transmission of a disease: the agent, the host, and the environment.

Agent

At the center of the KFD triad lies the agent, the Kyasanur Forest Disease Virus [KFDV]. KFDV is related closely to the Alkhurma virus. This belongs to the flavivirus genus, a group of single-stranded RNA viruses approximately 25 nm in diameter notorious for causing hemorrhagic fevers. KFDV's genetic makeup, with a genome of around 10.1 kilobases, shares similarities with other tick-borne flaviviruses, such as Alkhurma hemorrhagic fever virus and Omsk hemorrhagic fever virus. KFDV is a single polyprotein-encoding virus with a positive-sense RNA genome. Its polyprotein is divided post-translationally into structurally similar proteins.

C, E, and M, and seven proteins that are not structural [NS1 to NS5 with subdivisions in NS2a, NS2b, and NS4a, NS4b] are produced by post-translational cleavage of this polyprotein. Understanding the properties and behavior of this agent is vital for developing strategies to combat KFD.

Host

The second vertex of the triad is the host, the organism that harbors and can potentially transmit the disease. In the case of KFD, small mammals, notably monkeys, serve as the primary hosts for KFDV. These animals act as a natural reservoir for the virus, carrying it without always showing signs of illness. Various small organisms that inhabit forests, such as shrews, rodents, insectivorous bats, and numerous birds, play a crucial role in maintaining the virus's enzootic cycle within the forest environment. Wild monkeys, such as bonnet monkeys [*Macaca radiata*] and langurs with black faces [*Semnopithecus entellus*], contract the virus through tick bites and are highly inclined to infection. People are inadvert hosts of dead ends. Cattle play a crucial role in maintaining tick populations. The family Ixodidae [Hard Ticks], particularly the genus *Haemaphysalis*, serves as both a vector of the virus and a reservoir. Key tick species transmitting KFD include *H. turturis, Haemaphysalis spinigera, H. kinneari, H. kyasaurensis, H. wellingtoni, H. papuana, H. cuspidata, H. minuta, Dermacentor auratus, Ixodes petauristae,* and *H. bispinosa*. Ticks depend entirely on sucking blood to survive. They are external parasites that feed on mammals, birds, and reptiles. The primary vectors, ticks of the genus *Haemaphysalis*, include *H. spinigera* and *H. turturis*, which inhabit forest vegetation and infest numerous small mammals and birds. Humans typically become infected by biting unfed nymphal ticks, which are more human-centered than mature ticks. KFDV is transmitted from infected larvae to nymphs and adults, maintaining transovarial and transstadial transmission within the ecosystem.

On the other hand, humans are considered accidental hosts and are infected through the bite of an infected tick or, in rare cases, contact with infected animal tissues or fluids. Identifying susceptible hosts is crucial for understanding how the virus circulates and for targeting prevention efforts effectively.

Environment

The final part of the triad is the environment, the surrounding conditions that influence the interaction between the agent and the host. KFD is endemic, meaning it is constantly present and locally restricted in the southwestern region of India, particularly the Western Ghats Forest ecosystem. This specific environment provides a suitable habitat for the *Haemaphysalis spinigera*, the hard tick that is the primary vector for transmitting KFDV between wildlife and humans. The presence of this tick vector and the more susceptible animal hosts in this environment contribute significantly to the persistence and transmission of KFDV.

By examining KFD through the lens of the epidemiological triad, valuable insights into the disease's ecology can be gained. This helps us understand that KFDV exploits susceptible small mammal hosts and the KFD-endemic environment to infect accidental human hosts through tick bites. This knowledge is essential for developing effective control strategies. By targeting the KFDV agent through vaccines or antiviral medications, managing the tick vector population through acaricides [tick control agents], and educating communities about the risks in KFD-endemic areas, one can disrupt the triad and significantly reduce the threat of KFD.

Epidemiology

The story of Kyasanur Forest Disease [KFD] began dramatically in 1957. Scientists investigating unwell and fallen monkeys in the Kyasanur Forest faced a new threat. It turned out that these monkeys were infected with a previously unknown virus. During the investigation, scientists and local forest workers were bitten by infected ticks, resulting in a hemorrhagic illness. This initial outbreak marked the beginning of KFD in humans. Over 466 cases were reported that year, followed by another 181 the next. The disease predominantly affects young adults who enter forested areas during the dry season. Since its discovery, KFD has caused epidemic outbreaks, affecting anywhere from 100 to 500 people annually. KFD can be quite severe, with a case mortality rate ranging from two to ten percentage [23].

KFDV: Not Just an Indian Story

Isolated cases of KFDV were suspected in Saudi Arabia and China. This suggests the virus might have a more comprehensive geographical presence than initially thought.

Alkhurma Subgroup: In Saudi Arabia, a variant called the Alkhurma subgroup emerged during the mid-1990s. Interestingly, despite a geographical separation of about 4,000 km and a gap of nearly 40 years, this variant showed a high degree of similarity [only 8% difference] to the Indian reference strain.

Initially identified as the Nanjianyin virus, this virus was found in China in 1989 and is currently recognized as a KFDV strain.

However, there is some uncertainty about its authenticity due to its close resemblance to the Indian strain from 1957.

Spread and Mode of Transmission of KFD

KFD transmission is *via* the bite of an infected hard tick, particularly the *Haemaphysalis spinigera* species. By feeding on human blood, these ticks transmit the virus to people that they have contracted from infected animals. They serve as a reservoir for the virus in the environment and are carriers for extended periods.

While less common, KFD can also spread through direct contact with infected animals, especially monkeys, which are the primary hosts for the virus. This can happen if you handle sick or dead monkeys or come into contact with their bodily fluids. It is essential to avoid contact with wildlife in areas endemic to KFD.

Humans are the Kyasanur Forest Disease Virus's accidental and terminal hosts [KFDV], primarily contracting the virus through the bite of nymphal stage ticks. Exposure to tick bites often occurs during activities, such as handling monkey carcasses, visiting forests for agricultural purposes, collecting dry wood, cattle grazing, or engaging in recreational activities. Significant factors associated with KFD include:

• Handling cattle.
• Frequent forest visits for livelihood.
• The home's compound is filled with heaps of dried leaves.

The most affected animal species, *Macaca radiata* and *Semnopithecus entellus,* act as sentinels for KFDV spread. Between 1957 and 2020, over 3,314 deaths of monkeys linked to KFD were reported from the endemic zones of the Western Ghats. When KFDV-infected monkeys die, ticks drop off their bodies, creating "hot spots." A fifty-foot radius from the location of a monkey's unusual death is considered a hot spot. These deaths signal the beginning of an epidemic or a potential human outbreak.

Several environmental factors play a role in KFD outbreaks. Warmer temperatures, higher humidity, and suitable tick habitats [like tall grasses and forests] all contribute to increased tick activity. Additionally, the movement of infected animals, notably monkeys, into human settlements can bring the virus closer to people, raising the risk of exposure.

The epidemic period for KFD typically starts in October or November, peaks from January to April, and slows down by May and June. This period corresponds to the high activity of nymphal ticks from November to May. The highest number of monkey deaths also starts from December to May, aligning with the nymph stage of the ticks. There have been no reports of person-to-person transmission of KFD, though laboratory-acquired infections were noted in the early days of virus discovery due to inadequate containment facilities [24].

Indian Scenario of KFD

While Kyasanur Forest Disease [KFD] is primarily associated with Karnataka, the virus has unfortunately recently spread to neighboring states. The following is a timeline of outbreaks in these regions:

Tamil Nadu [2012-2013]

KFD reached Tamil Nadu's Nilgiri district, where the virus was detected in dead monkeys during autopsies. Notably, no human cases were reported during this period, and prompt vaccination efforts likely contributed to preventing an outbreak. However, a single human case did surface in 2016.

Kerala [2013-2015]

KFD made its presence known in Kerala as well. While only six human cases emerged in 2013-2014, a significant outbreak unfolded in 2014-2015, resulting in 102 confirmed cases and, tragically, 11 deaths.

Goa [2015-2016]

Goa also faced a KFD outbreak in the North Goa district from 2015 to 2016. Fortunately, the scale was smaller compared to Kerala, with 36 human cases and one death reported.

Maharashtra [2016]

The neighboring state of Maharashtra was not spared either. An outbreak erupted in the Sindhudurg district in 2016, with a significant number of cases [129] and fatalities [8].

KFD Status in Karnataka

KFD was first identified in 1957 in Karnataka and remains the disease's epicenter in India. The disease is indigenous to the Western Ghats region of Karnataka, with regular outbreaks reported from Shivamogga district, Uttara Kannada, Dakshina Kannada, and Chikkamagaluru.

In recent years, the geographical distribution of KFD has elaborated, with cases reported from neighboring states like Goa, Kerala, Tamil Nadu, and Maharashtra. This expansion is attributed to increased human-animal interactions, climate change, and improved disease surveillance and reporting [NCDC 218].

Haemaphysalis spinigera

This tick species is the reason for spreading KFD among animals and humans. Birds and cattle serve as hosts for these vector ticks. While all stages of *H. spinigera* can feed on humans, only infected nymphs transmit KFD through their bites. The virus is not passed by transovarial transmission. Other *Haemaphysalis* species, like *Haemaphysalis turturis*, also contribute to the KFD cycle in animals. The virus has even been found in 14 different tick species, including *Haemaphysalis*, *Ixodes*, *and Dermacentor*, highlighting the complex transmission web.

The tick species *Haemaphysalis spinigera* inhabits forests, where its larvae and nymphs feed on various tiny forest creatures, birds, and monkeys. This species' adult ticks heavily parasitize cattle, contributing to the growth of the parasite population. In the KFD region, *H. spinigera* ticks are most frequently discovered on plants and in ground drags. This species is commonly found in southern, central, and northern India, as well as in the dense and evergreen tropical forests of Sri Lanka.

Life Cycle of *Haemaphysalis spinigera*

The two body parts of *Haemaphysalis spinigera*, an arachnid, are a united head, thorax, and abdomen. Tick adults have four sets of legs with no wings or antennae. Complete metamorphosis occurs during the arachnid life cycle, in which eggs hatch into nymphs that look like adults. During the enzootic phase, the virus is transmitted mainly by tick species, particularly *H. spinigera*, and small animals, including rats, mice, shrews, porcupines, squirrels, and rodents. Bats and birds are less important hosts in comparison. Humans do not aid in the spread of viruses; instead, they are accidental hosts. Human activities like grazing, clearing land for building, and other agricultural operations upset the previously steady enzootic state. Tick populations skyrocketed as cattle were brought in to graze close to the forest, giving ticks a fresh and plentiful supply of blood meals. Cattle are essential to the survival of tick populations, although they are not involved in the virus's maintenance. Infection hotspots are produced when monkeys come into contact with infected ticks, which causes the monkeys to become sick, spread, and transmit the virus. Monkeys are known to be the virus's amplifying hosts because they display severe viremia, a condition that can be lethal. Epizootics in monkeys, namely the South Indian bonnet macaque [*Macaca radiata*] and *Presbytis entellus*- the black-faced langur, are linked to seasonal outbreaks of KFD.

The life cycle of ticks begins as eggs [stage I], which then hatch into six-legged larvae [stage II]. After a week or so of feeding on small animals, monkeys, or birds, these larvae separate and molt into eight-legged nymphs [stage III]. After feeding on people or other animals for three to eleven days, nymphs separate and molt into adult ticks, which are either male or female, around one month later, depending on the environment. Adult ticks use their legs to feel and seek prey by utilizing Haller's organs to detect heat and carbon dioxide on their first pair of legs. They climb grass and plants. Ticks latch onto warm-blooded animals as they pass, protrude their mouths, and feed on blood [stage IV]. Tick saliva may infiltrate the host's circulation during feeding, which might result in the transmission of KFDV. Ticks usually mate on the host, male or female. A few weeks later, the engorged female separates and deposits 1,000–8,000 eggs on a leaf. Before they die, ticks typically have a lifespan of one year.

Bionomics

The region where Kyasanur Forest Disease [KFD] is prevalent is a patchwork of different habitats, each with its unique characteristics:

Forestry Mosaic

The landscape combines forests, cultivated valleys, and grasslands, creating a diverse ecological tapestry.

Forest Focus

Forests are vital, providing essential resources for living organisms [biotic] and the non-living environment [abiotic]. These forests are categorized into three main types: semi-evergreen, semi-deciduous, and deciduous, often blending into one another in neighboring areas. Forest borders with grasslands usually have transition zones of shrubs or thickets. Grasslands themselves may contain dense clumps of vegetation.

A study revealed variations in tick populations across these different habitats. *H. turturis* and *H. kinneari* are the dominant tick species in semi-deciduous and evergreen forests. The number of *H. spinigera* and *H. turturis* nymphs [immature ticks] also varies depending on the local animal life and ecological conditions. Unlike most other tick species in the KFD area, *H. spinigera* feeds primarily on cattle. This makes them more common in deciduous forests and plantations [teak and eucalyptus] where cattle graze.

This knowledge of the KFD-endemic area's diverse habitats and tick distribution is crucial. It helps us identify areas with a higher KFD transmission risk and more effectively target preventive measures [25]

Clinical Features of KFD

Kyasanur Forest Disease [KFD] usually manifests as a biphasic sickness following 3 to 8 days of incubation. The symptoms appear suddenly and include chills, a maximum temperature of about 40°C, or 104°F, sensitivity to light, and a frontal headache. This is followed by a persistent fever lasting 12 days or longer. Vomiting, diarrhea, coughing, severe pain in the lower back, neck, and limbs, as well as acute prostration, are frequently experienced during this time. A papulovesicular eruption on the soft palate is a significant diagnostic indicator in certain patients. Additional typical symptoms, *i.e.*, blood in the stools, spitting up blood [hemoptysis], bleeding from the mouth and nostrils [epistaxis], and gastrointestinal bleeding leading to black feces [melena]. The healing period following the start of Kyasanur Forest Disease [KFD] is called the convalescent phase, lasting up to four weeks on average. A recurrence of symptoms often lasts for two to twelve days and happens one to two weeks following the initial febrile phase. The same symptoms as the previous phase are present throughout this relapse phase, along with possible new ones, such as mental problems, vertigo, and aberrant reflexes. Hematological characteristics of consistently present KFD include leucopenia [a decrease in total leukocytes] and thrombocytopenia. Intra-alveolar hemorrhage, or bleeding into the lungs, and extensive gastrointestinal hemorrhage, which may be fatal due to subsequent infections, are examples of terminal consequences [26].

There are four phases to this biphasic sickness, and each one lasts around one week:

Stage I: With symptoms including hypotension, sore throat, diarrhea, vomiting, hepatomegaly, anorexia, insomnia, severe pain in the upper and lower extremities, and prostration, the first prodromal stage starts with a sudden onset of fever and severe headache. During the 1st or 2nd infection, bradycardia and conjunctival inflammation are often seen, along with acute lymphopenia and eosinopenia.

Stage II: Hematemesis, black stools [melena], blood in the stool, and sporadic nosebleeds [epistaxis] are among the hemorrhagic consequences that define stage II. Neurological symptoms, such as tremors, odd reflexes, and mental disorientation, are also noted. In certain instances, a coma may set in just before death, or bronchopneumonia may develop.

Stages III and IV: Some patients may have a feverish last phase after recovery.

While fever is a hallmark symptom, KFD can lead to more serious issues. A possible outcome is parenchymal degeneration, which causes harm to vital organs of the kidneys and liver. Hemorrhagic pneumonitis, a condition causing lung bleeding, can occur in some cases. The body's immune system goes into overdrive, with a marked increase in specific cells [reticuloendothelial elements] in the liver and spleen. This hyperactive response can be harmful. A process called erythrophagocytosis, where immune cells inappropriately engulf red blood cells, can also be observed in some patients.

These clinical manifestations highlight the potential severity of KFD. The virus can impact not just a single system but wreak havoc on multiple organs, causing bleeding, organ damage, and an overzealous immune response [27]

High-risk Groups/ Factors

Kyasanur Forest Disease [KFD] poses a particular threat to specific groups of people. Here is a breakdown of the high-risk categories:

Forest Dwellers

People living in KFD-endemic forest areas are constantly exposed to the environment where the virus thrives.

Occupational Exposure

People whose jobs involve direct or indirect contact with ticks are at higher risk.

This includes:

- Forestry workers [guards, rangers, watchers]
- Plantation workers [coffee, tea, cashew nut, *etc.*]
- Farmers working near forests
- Forest department officials
- Tourists and wildlife photographers
- Shepherds

- Firewood and dry leaf collectors
- Hunters
- Communities of tribes residing in forested places
- Cashew nut and areca nut farm workers
- Individuals who handle dead animal carcasses
- Campers who travel through forests

Cattle Connection

People who handle cattle and frequent KFD-endemic forests are at a significantly higher risk than those who do not.

Seasonal Spike

KFD cases tend to rise in the withered season, typically between June and November, with a peak from March to December.

Forest Activities

Areas with combined forest-plantation activities, incredibly dense, moist, evergreen forests, and high cattle populations create a higher KFD risk environment.

Risky Practices

Collecting and storing firewood and dry leaves near homes and using dry leaves as cattle bedding can increase exposure to infected ticks.

Handling Dead Monkeys

This is a hazardous activity, as monkeys are primary hosts for the KFD virus.

By understanding these risk factors, individuals and communities can take steps to protect themselves from KFD [28].

Diagnosis of KFD

Historically, KFD was diagnosed by inoculating patient serum into *Swiss albino* or suckling mice, followed by serological tests like hemagglutination inhibition, neutralization tests, and complement fixation. However, modern diagnostic approaches have shifted towards more effective molecular-based techniques. These include:

- RT-PCR assays, such as TaqMan-based RT-PCR, simple RT-PCR, and nested RT-PCR
- Detection of IgM and IgG antibodies using Enzyme-Linked Immunosorbent Assay [ELISA]

These molecular methods target the highly conserved NS-5 gene sequence within the Flavivirus genus, allowing for accurate and rapid diagnosis of KFD [29].

Treatment

For KFD, there is no particular antiviral medication. Management of the disease is primarily supportive, focusing on the alleviation of symptoms and the prevention of complications. Supportive care includes:

- Administration of fluids.
- Management of fever and pain.
- The monitoring and treatment of bleeding and neurological manifestations.

In severe cases, hospitalization and intensive care may be required. In rare instances, the antiviral medication ribavirin has been employed, but its efficacy in treating KFD is still under investigation [30].

Climate's Influence on KFD: A Look at Environmental Factors and their Impact

The relevance of climate change has peaked, influencing the evolving epidemiology of Kyasanur Forest Disease [KFD]. Changes in precipitation patterns and temperature directly affect the survival, development, and behavior of the tick vectors responsible for transmitting KFDV, as well as the distribution and availability of their animal hosts.

Research indicates that *Haemaphysalis spinigera*, the principal vector of KFDV, thrives in warm and humid conditions. Increasing temperatures and alterations in rainfall patterns can create favorable environments for the tick's reproduction and survival, potentially expanding its geographic range and increasing human exposure.

Furthermore, the biphasic nature of KFD, characterized by a secondary wave of symptoms approximately three weeks after the initial onset, correlates with seasonal variations in tick activity. Peak incidences of KFD cases often coincide with drier and warmer months, when *Haemaphysalis spinigera* exhibits heightened activity and greater abundance.

Deforestation and Habitat Fragmentation

Deforestation and habitat fragmentation play crucial roles in the emergence and spread of Kyasanur Forest Disease [KFD]. The destruction of natural forest ecosystems disrupts the intricate balance among tick vectors, animal hosts, and human populations, facilitating increased contact and transmission of the virus.

The extensive deforestation in the Western Ghats and changes in land use have occurred in recent decades. These environmental changes have fragmented forest habitats, displacing and altering the movements of animal hosts like monkeys, which serve as natural reservoirs for KFDV.

As these animal hosts venture into human-dominated landscapes, the opportunities for human-animal interactions and subsequent virus transmission rise. Moreover, the degradation of forest habitats can affect the ecology of tick vectors, potentially altering their distribution and abundance.

Biodiversity Loss and Ecological Imbalance

A healthy ecosystem boasts a diverse range of small mammal species. These mammals act as alternative hosts for the KFD-carrying ticks. However, when biodiversity declines, these alternative hosts become less abundant. With fewer alternative hosts, the ticks rely more on the primary host – monkeys – for survival. This increased focus on monkeys leads to a phenomenon called host amplification, where the virus replicates more efficiently within the monkey population. This, in turn, increases the amount of virus circulating in the environment.

Predator Paradox: Predators play a crucial role in maintaining a healthy balance within an ecosystem. When predator populations decline due to habitat loss or other factors, rodent and small mammal populations can surge. These unchecked populations become additional reservoirs for the KFD virus, increasing the risk of spillover to humans.

Risky Encounters

The food chain disruption and ecological imbalance can also lead to more frequent interactions between humans and KFD-infected animals. This raises the chances of people coming into contact with the virus, either directly through animal encounters or indirectly through infected tick bites [31].

Seasonal Fluctuations

While some tick species maintain a year-round presence with minor fluctuations, *Haemaphysalis* species exhibit distinct seasonal dominance:

October to December: This period is prime time for larvae, the immature stage of the tick.

January to May: The spotlight shifts to nymphs, the next stage in the tick's life cycle.

June to September: Adults take center stage during these months [32].

KFD in Shivamogga: A Seasonal Predicament

In Shivamogga district, Kyasanur Forest Disease [KFD] follows a predictable pattern with the seasons, with a recurring annual pattern of cases observed between 2011 and 2018. Here is a breakdown of this seasonal cycle:

Start: KFD cases typically begin to emerge in January, marking the start of the transmission season.

Peakness: By March, the number of cases reaches its peak. This coincides with the dry season in the region, when animals are forced to congregate near limited water sources, increasing their chances of encountering infected ticks.

Gradual Decline: After the peak in March, KFD cases start to decline gradually.

Low Transmission Period: By June or July, the number of cases dips significantly, reaching near zero. This period of low transmission usually lasts until October.

November Resurgence: As November arrives, KFD cases reappear, marking a new cycle's start.

A Seven-Month Window: Overall, the window for KFD transmission in Shivamogga district is limited to a maximum of seven months, typically spanning from November to May. This seasonal pattern highlights the critical role of environmental factors, particularly the dry season, in influencing KFD outbreaks [33].

Why Does Seasonality Matter?

The seasonal pattern of tick prevalence has significant implications for the transmission of KFD.

Aligned with Transmission Window: The peak season for nymphs [January to May] coincides with the dry season in KFD-endemic areas. This dry season forces animals to congregate around limited water sources, increasing the chances of encountering infected ticks.

Higher Risk for Humans: Nymphs are the primary life stage of *Haemaphysalis* ticks that transmit KFD to humans. Their peak activity during the dry season overlaps with increased human outdoor activity, raising the risk of tick bites and potential KFD infection (Fig. **3**).

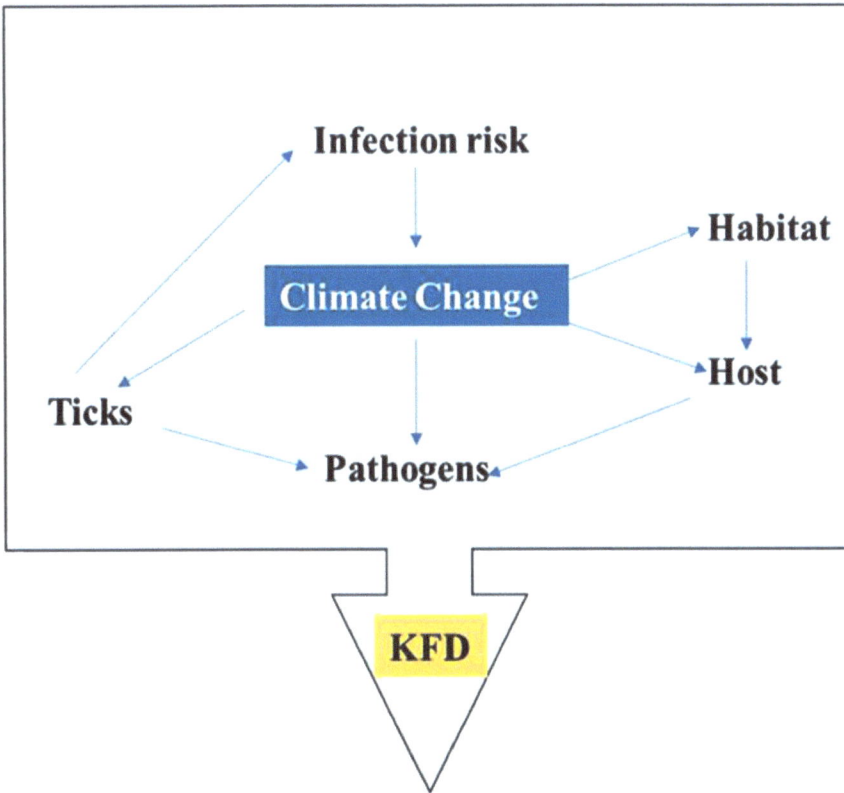

Fig. (3). Climate change as an influential factor for KFD transmission.

Climate Change Data on KFD in Recent Years

India's temperature increased by 0.60°C between 1951 and 2010, according to thorough research by the Indian Ministry of Earth Science. In states like Karnataka, Kerala, Goa, and Maharashtra, where KFD is endemic, this temperature increase was especially notable. The life cycle of tick vectors, especially the main KFD vector *Haemaphysalis spinigera*, may be accelerated by rising temperatures. Like most ectotherms, ticks are extremely sensitive to temperature fluctuations; higher temperatures can improve their ability to spread the virus, increase blood feed frequency, and speed reproduction. According to a study conducted by Pramanik *et al.* in Southern India, researchers identified key bioclimatic variables influencing the distribution of *Haemaphysalis spinigera*. The study found that the warmest quarter temperature ranged from 25.4 to 30°C, and the diurnal temperature varied between 8 and 10°C, as determined using the MaxEnt model.

Concurrently, precipitation patterns have changed significantly in KFD-affected areas, with annual precipitation levels in Maharashtra, Goa, Karnataka, and Kerala declining by −0.71 mm, −3.82 mm, −0.05 mm, and −1.43 mm, respectively. These rainfall declines upset the natural equilibrium of forested areas, affecting tick populations and their interactions with rodents, monkeys, and humans. Additionally, decreased precipitation is linked to drier environmental conditions during specific seasons, which may prolong tick activity by establishing favorable microclimates in the forest floor and leaf litter.

Rising temperatures and decreasing rainfall significantly affect the spread of KFD in areas like the Western Ghats, where the illness is most common. Heavy rains during the monsoon season [June to October] might temporarily wash away or decrease nymphal tick activity. Tick populations may be able to multiply more quickly and continue their activity over the next dry season if precipitation decreases and irregular rainfall patterns restrict this natural confinement mechanism (Fig. **4**).

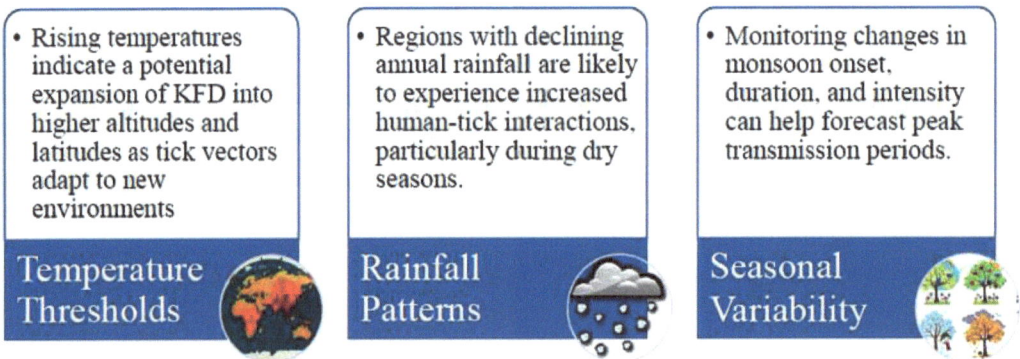

- Rising temperatures indicate a potential expansion of KFD into higher altitudes and latitudes as tick vectors adapt to new environments

- Regions with declining annual rainfall are likely to experience increased human-tick interactions, particularly during dry seasons.

- Monitoring changes in monsoon onset, duration, and intensity can help forecast peak transmission periods.

Temperature Thresholds   Rainfall Patterns   Seasonal Variability

Fig. (4). Climate data as predictors of epidemiological shifts.

Mathematical Models with Examples for Climate Change's Impact on KFD

Mathematical models are an effective tool to investigate and forecast how climate change affects the epidemiology of KFD. These models incorporate human interactions, vector and host ecology, and climatic factors, such as temperature and precipitation. A next-generation matrix modeling framework was developed to understand the transmission dynamics and host contributions to tick-borne diseases, focusing on Kyasanur Forest Disease Virus [KFD] across various habitats. The study highlighted the significant roles of transovarial transmission, small mammals, and birds in maintaining KFD, challenging prior assumptions about primates. Habitat variation may influence disease risk, but further research is needed to confirm this. Key knowledge gaps and research priorities are outlined to guide interventions and control efforts [34]. Some of the real-world examples are as follows:

SIR [Susceptible-Infectious-Recovered] Model for KFD

The SIR model accounts for how susceptible individuals [S] interact with infectious individuals [I], and eventually recover [R], with climate variables modifying transmission rates.

The SIR model categorizes the population into three groups: susceptible, infectious, and recovered. In the context of KFD, these models have been adapted to include vector and host populations, while incorporating climate variables, such as temperature and rainfall. For example, in the Shivamogga district of Karnataka, where KFD is endemic, SIR models have been used to simulate outbreaks by analyzing seasonal changes in vector [tick] populations. Studies found that post-monsoon temperature increases and reduced rainfall significantly enhance the transmission of the KFD virus by increasing human exposure to infected ticks during dry months. These models have also shown how targeted interventions, such as pre-emptive vaccination campaigns during high-risk months, can effectively reduce cases [35].

Climate-Driven Vector-Host Models

Vector-host models simulate interactions between tick vectors, wildlife hosts [*e.g.*, monkeys and rodents], and human populations. These models explicitly include climate-driven factors that influence tick activity, such as vegetation cover, temperature thresholds, and precipitation. In Goa, where KFD outbreaks have become more frequent, a climate-driven vector-host model demonstrated how heavy monsoon rains create ideal tick breeding environments by increasing vegetation density. The dry season that follows forces host species, such as monkeys, to migrate closer to human settlements, thereby increasing human-tick interactions. This model highlights the role of seasonal rainfall patterns in shaping the disease's epidemiology and provides a basis for early warning systems in areas with similar ecological conditions.

Spatial-Temporal Models

Spatial-temporal models explore the geographic spread of KFD over time, considering environmental changes and human activities. These models are particularly useful for understanding the expanding range of KFD into new areas, likely driven by deforestation and rising temperatures. For instance, in Karnataka, spatial modeling predicted the movement of KFD into higher altitudes as warming temperatures allowed tick vectors to establish themselves in previously cooler regions. These models also identified Uttara Kannada and Chikkamagaluru as emerging hotspots due to a combination of deforestation and increasing human encroachment into forested areas. Such insights help authorities allocate resources for vaccination and surveillance in vulnerable regions [35].

Threshold-Based Models

This model defines outbreak conditions based on climate-driven changes to the basic reproduction number [R_0]. It represents the average number of secondary infections caused by a single infected individual. When $R_0 > 1$, an outbreak is likely to occur. For KFD, these models incorporate climate factors, vector population dynamics, and human behavior.

In Kerala, researchers employed a threshold model to investigate KFD outbreaks in Wayanad. They discovered that warmer temperatures above 25°C enhanced the survival and reproduction rates of ticks, while cumulative rainfall below 500 mm during the dry season increased human exposure to infected ticks. These findings informed targeted vaccination programs and awareness campaigns, thereby reducing the disease burden in high-risk areas.

Agent-Based Models

Agent-based models simulate the behavior of individual agents [*e.g.*, humans, ticks, monkeys] in a virtual environment, considering their interactions with each other and the environment. These models are ideal for capturing the complex dynamics of KFD transmission, which involves multiple hosts, vectors, and climatic variables. In a study conducted in the Western Ghats, agent-based models revealed how the migration patterns of bonnet macaques [a primary host for KFD] are influenced by habitat fragmentation and food scarcity during the dry season. These models also showed that human-tick interactions increase near water sources during dry months, aligning with observed seasonal peaks in KFD cases. This approach provides granular insights into the spatial and temporal dynamics of KFD transmission, aiding in the design of site-specific control measures.

Machine Learning Models

Machine learning models, such as Random Forest and Support Vector Machines, analyze large datasets to identify patterns and predict outbreaks. These models incorporate variables, such as temperature, rainfall, vegetation indices, and historical case data, to make accurate predictions.

For example, a Random Forest model trained on historical outbreak data in Karnataka identified declining annual rainfall and rising temperatures as key predictors of KFD incidence. The model successfully forecasted high-risk zones for the 2021 transmission season, enabling health officials to implement timely interventions. Such models are particularly useful for developing real-time surveillance systems and guiding public health responses.

Integrated Climate-Epidemiology Models

Integrated models combine multiple approaches to provide a holistic understanding of KFD dynamics. These models incorporate climate projections, vector ecology, host population dynamics, and human behavior to forecast long-term trends in disease distribution. A study in Goa demonstrated how integrated models could predict the impact of climate change on KFD transmission over the next decade. The models projected that rising temperatures and shifting rainfall patterns would extend the transmission season and expand the disease's geographic range into previously unaffected areas. These findings underscore the need for adaptive public health strategies that address the long-term impacts of climate change [36].

Applications of Mathematical Models

Outbreak Prediction

In Karnataka, SIR and threshold-based models helped predict seasonal peaks in KFD cases, guiding vaccination schedules and resource allocation.

Hotspot Identification

Spatial-temporal and machine learning models identified emerging hotspots in Uttara Kannada and Chikkamagaluru, enabling targeted interventions.

Policy Development

Integrated models informed the development of long-term strategies to address the impact of climate change on KFD transmission.

Surveillance Optimization

Climate-driven models guided the placement of tick traps and wildlife monitoring efforts, improving the efficiency of surveillance programs.

To conclude, mathematical models play a crucial role in understanding and mitigating the impact of climate change on KFD. By incorporating climate variables and ecological data, these models provide actionable insights into disease dynamics, enabling targeted interventions and informed policy decisions. As climate change continues to reshape the epidemiology of vector-borne diseases, the use of advanced modeling techniques will become increasingly important in safeguarding public health.

To effectively address the challenges posed by KFD in the context of a changing climate, it is crucial to bridge the insights provided by mathematical models with practical intervention strategies. The integration of predictive modeling with ground-level measures ensures a comprehensive approach to disease management. This alignment of predictive insights with actionable measures emphasizes the need for a proactive stance in combating KFD. Understanding the seasonal and ecological nuances of the disease provides a foundation for implementing targeted interventions that align with the cycles of vector and host activity. By leveraging this knowledge, public health officials can optimize their efforts and enhance the effectiveness of control measures [36].

Understanding the Cycle for Better Control

Knowing this seasonal trend is a valuable tool for public health officials. By anticipating the KFD season, they can implement preventive measures more effectively. This might involve:

Intensified Tick Control Efforts: Focusing tick control efforts during the peak nymphal activity period [which coincides with the peak KFD season] can significantly reduce tick populations and the risk of transmission.

Targeted Awareness Campaigns: Educating communities about KFD risk factors and preventive measures during the high-risk season can empower them to protect themselves from tick bites.

Resource Allocation: Strategic allocation of healthcare resources to prepare for the influx of KFD cases during the peak season can ensure a more efficient response to the outbreak.

Surveillance and Monitoring Strategies

Death Surveillance of Monkeys

An essential part of the monitoring system is tracking the mortality of monkeys in KFD-endemic regions, as this information may indicate possible outbreaks before they occur. The creation of a reporting system, the gathering and transportation of monkey samples, and the examination of these samples for the presence of KFDV are all covered under the operational guidelines for the surveillance of monkey death.

Vector Monitoring

Tick populations in endemic locations, especially those of the *Haemaphysalis spinigera* species, are the main focus of vector surveillance for KFD. This entails determining suitable sample regions, bringing tick collecting and identification techniques into practice, and checking tick pools for the presence of KFDV.

Environmental Observation

Recognizing how climate change and other environmental factors affect the ecological variables and the epidemiology of the illness depends on integrating environmental monitoring into the KFD surveillance system. This might involve keeping an eye on the weather, precipitation, and temperature in addition to evaluating habitat fragmentation and changes in land use.

To detect high-risk locations and anticipate possible outbreaks, integrating Geographic Information Systems [GIS] with remote sensing can benefit environmental data's spatial and temporal analysis [37].

Mitigation and Control Strategies

Immunization and Vaccination

One of the most critical aspects of the disease management plan is creating and implementing an efficient KFD vaccination. To guard against the disease, the formalin-inactivated virus-based KFD vaccine has been administered in India's endemic areas.

Several vaccines were investigated for the management of the illness until the inactivated [formalin] KFD Virus [KFDV] vaccine that is presently in use was created in chick embryo fibroblasts. These included a live attenuated vaccination by repeated tissue culture passages, a formalin-inactivated vaccine from mice brain, a 5–10% solution of the Russian Spring-Summer Encephalitis [RSSE] virus, and a tissue culture source. After receiving two doses of the formalized KFDV vaccine, 59% of the participants in field experiments conducted in 1970–71 showed a serological response.

In light of changing climatic conditions, immunization is still one of the critical strategies for lowering the burden of KFD. Therefore, efforts to increase the vaccine's effectiveness, safety, and accessibility are ongoing.

Vector Management Techniques

Controlling vectors that aim to eliminate the *Haemaphysalis spinigera* tick is crucial to reducing the effects of environmental variables and climate change on spreading KFD. This might involve promoting personal preventive measures among high-risk communities, using acaricides, and implementing tick-borne illness management strategies.

Furthermore, the creation of innovative vector control techniques, including the use of biological control agents or the interruption of tick life cycles, may present viable paths for resolving the issues caused by climate change.

Conservation of Biodiversity and Restoration of Habitats

The influence of environmental variables on the epidemiology of KFD can be significantly reduced by initiatives to repair and protect the natural ecosystems in endemic regions of the disease. This may involve promoting ecological balance, safeguarding biodiversity, and implementing sustainable forest management techniques.

The danger of human-animal contact and the possibility of viral transmission may be decreased by preserving the integrity of natural ecosystems, which helps to manage and avoid Kyasanur forest disease overall [38].

CONCLUSION

Climate change profoundly influences the ecology and epidemiology of vector-borne diseases like Kyasanur Forest Disease. Understanding these dynamics is essential for predicting and mitigating future outbreaks. Effective surveillance, integrated vector control strategies, and public awareness campaigns are crucial for managing the impact of KFD in the context of changing climate conditions. Continued research into the interactions between climate change, tick biology, and disease transmission dynamics is needed to develop adaptive strategies and safeguard public health in endemic regions.

REFERENCES

[1]   Kilpatrick AM, Randolph SE. Drivers, dynamics, and control of emerging vector-borne zoonotic diseases. Glob Health Impacts Vector-Borne Dis 2016. Available from: https://www.ncbi.nlm.nih.gov/books/NBK390427/

[2]   Horefti E. The importance of the one health concept in combating zoonoses. Pathogens 2023; 12(8): 977.
[http://dx.doi.org/10.3390/pathogens12080977] [PMID: 37623937]

[3]   Bisen P, Raghuvanshi R. Kyasanur Forest Disease. 2013; pp. 361-74.
[http://dx.doi.org/10.1002/9781118393277.ch13]

[4]   Burton E. Module 102: General anatomy of hard ticks 2021. Available from: https://pressbooks.umn.edu/cvdl/chapter/module-10-2-ticks/

[5]   Kopsco HL, Gronemeyer P, Mateus-Pinilla N, Smith RL. Current and future habitat suitability models for four ticks of medical concern in illinois, USA. Insects 2023; 14(3): 213.
[http://dx.doi.org/10.3390/insects14030213] [PMID: 36975898]

[6]   Chakraborty S, Andrade FCD, Ghosh S, Uelmen J, Ruiz MO. Historical expansion of kyasanur forest disease in India From 1957 to 2017: A retrospective analysis. Geohealth 2019; 3(2): 44-55.
[http://dx.doi.org/10.1029/2018GH000164] [PMID: 32159030]

[7]   Coons LB, Rothschild M. Ticks. In: Capinera JL, Ed. Encyclopedia of entomology. Dordrecht: Springer Netherlands 2008; pp. 3775-801. Acari: Ixodida [Internet]
[http://dx.doi.org/10.1007/978-1-4020-6359-6_2457]

[8]   Sonenshine D, Roe RM. External and internal anatomy of ticks. Biol Ticks 2014; 2: 74-98.

[9]   Sonenshine DE. Ticks. In: Resh VH, Cardé RT, Eds. Encyclopedia of Insects. San Diego: Academic Press 2009; pp. 1003-11. [Second Edition] [Internet] Available from: https://www.sciencedirect.com/science/article/pii/B9780123741448002642
[http://dx.doi.org/10.1016/B978-0-12-374144-8.00264-2]

[10]   Nava S, Venzal JM, González-Acuña D, Martins TF, Guglielmone AA. Chapter 255 - Ticks. In: Resh VH, Cardé RT, editors. Encyclopedia of Insects 2nd Edition. San Diego: Academic Press, 2024. Available from: https://www.sciencedirect.com/science/article/pii/B9780128110751000017

[11]   Silaghi C. Prevalence and genetic analysis of Anaplasma phagocytophilum and Spotted Fever Group rickettsiae in the tick Ixodes ricinus in urban and periurban sites in southern Germany 2008.
[http://dx.doi.org/DOI: 10.5282/edoc.9036]

[12]   Basu AK, Charles RA. Chapter 1 - A general account of ticks. Ticks of Trinidad and Tobago - an overview 2017; 1-33. Available from: https://www.sciencedirect.com/science/article/pii/B9780128097441000013

[13]   Firdisa Duguma M. International Journal of Advanced Multidisciplinary Research Review on identification of ixodidae tick species on bovine in and around Shanan Dhugo district, Eastern Ethiopia. Int J Multidiscip Res Rev 2022; 9: 202.

[14]   Balasubramanian R, Yadav PD, Sahina S, Nadh VA. The species distribution of ticks & the prevalence of Kyasanur forest disease virus in questing nymphal ticks from Western Ghats of Kerala, South India. Indian J Med Res 2021; 154(5): 743-9.
[http://dx.doi.org/10.4103/ijmr.IJMR_234_19] [PMID: 35532592]

[15]   Nuttall PA. Climate change impacts on ticks and tick-borne infections. Biologia (Bratisl) 2022; 77(6): 1503-12. [Bratisl].
[http://dx.doi.org/10.1007/s11756-021-00927-2]

[16]   Gilbert L, Aungier J, Tomkins JL. Climate of origin affects tick (*Ixodes ricinus*) host-seeking behavior in response to temperature: implications for resilience to climate change? Ecol Evol 2014; 4(7): 1186-98.

[http://dx.doi.org/10.1002/ece3.1014] [PMID: 24772293]

[17]   Gilbert L. The impacts of climate change on ticks and tick-borne disease risk. Annu Rev Entomol 2021; 66: 373-88.
[http://dx.doi.org/10.1146/annurev-ento-052720-094533]

[18]   Macleod J. *Ixodes ricinus* in relation to its physical environment. Parasitology 1935; 27(4): 489-500.
[http://dx.doi.org/10.1017/S0031182000015420]

[19]   Wilson C, Gasmi S, Bourgeois AC, *et al.* Surveillance for *Ixodes scapularis* and *Ixodes pacificus* ticks and their associated pathogens in Canada, 2019. Can Commun Dis Rep 2022; 48(5): 208-18.
[http://dx.doi.org/10.14745/ccdr.v48i05a04] [PMID: 37325256]

[20]   Danielová V, Rudenko N, Daniel M, *et al.* Extension of Ixodes ricinus ticks and agents of tick-borne diseases to mountain areas in the Czech Republic. Int J Med Microbiol 2006; 296 (Suppl. 40): 48-53.
[http://dx.doi.org/10.1016/j.ijmm.2006.02.007] [PMID: 16545603]

[21]   Wu X, Duvvuri VR, Lou Y, Ogden NH, Pelcat Y, Wu J. Developing a temperature-driven map of the basic reproductive number of the emerging tick vector of Lyme disease Ixodes scapularis in Canada. J Theor Biol 2013; 319: 50-61.
[http://dx.doi.org/10.1016/j.jtbi.2012.11.014] [PMID: 23206385]

[22]   Shiji PV, Viswanath V, Sreekumar S, Sreejith R, Majeed A, Udayabhaskaran V. Kyasanur forest disease - First reported case in Kerala. J Assoc Physicians India 2016; 64(3): 90-1.
[PMID: 27731570]

[23]   Shah SZ, Jabbar B, Ahmed N, *et al.* Epidemiology, pathogenesis, and control of a tick-Borne disease-kyasanur forest disease: Current status and future directions. Front Cell Infect Microbiol 2018; 8: 149.
[http://dx.doi.org/10.3389/fcimb.2018.00149] [PMID: 29868505]

[24]   Saravu K, Chunduru K. Kyasanur forest disease: A review on the emerging infectious disease. Journal of Clinical Infectious Diseases Society 2023; 1(1): 5.
[http://dx.doi.org/10.4103/CIDS.CIDS_13_23]

[25]   Naren Babu N, Jayaram A, Hemanth Kumar H, *et al.* Spatial distribution of Haemaphysalis species ticks and human Kyasanur Forest Disease cases along the Western Ghats of India, 2017–2018. Exp Appl Acarol 2019; 77(3): 435-47.
[http://dx.doi.org/10.1007/s10493-019-00345-9] [PMID: 30809731]

[26]   Munivenkatappa A, Sahay RR, Yadav PD, Viswanathan R, Mourya DT. Clinical & epidemiological significance of Kyasanur forest disease. Indian J Med Res 2018; 148(2): 145-50.
[http://dx.doi.org/10.4103/ijmr.IJMR_688_17] [PMID: 30381537]

[27]   Pattnaik P. Kyasanur forest disease: an epidemiological view in India. Rev Med Virol 2006; 16(3): 151-65.
[http://dx.doi.org/10.1002/rmv.495] [PMID: 16710839]

[28]   Pramanik M, Singh P, Dhiman RC. Identification of bio-climatic determinants and potential risk areas for Kyasanur forest disease in Southern India using MaxEnt modelling approach. BMC Infect Dis 2021; 21(1): 1226.
[http://dx.doi.org/10.1186/s12879-021-06908-9] [PMID: 34876036]

[29]   Gladson V, Moosan H, Mathew S, P D. Clinical and laboratory diagnostic features of Kyasanur forest disease: A study from wayanad, South India. Cureus 2021; 13(12): e20194.
[http://dx.doi.org/10.7759/cureus.20194] [PMID: 35004016]

[30]   Gupta DN. kyasanur forest disease 2018.

[31]   Singh P, Kumar P, Dhiman RC. Kyasanur forest disease and climatic attributes in India. J Vector Borne Dis 2022; 59(1): 79-85.
[http://dx.doi.org/10.4103/0972-9062.331408] [PMID: 35708408]

[32]   Murhekar MV, Kasabi GS, Mehendale SM, Mourya DT, Yadav PD, Tandale BV. On the transmission

pattern of Kyasanur Forest disease (KFD) in India. Infect Dis Poverty 2015; 4(1): 37.
[http://dx.doi.org/10.1186/s40249-015-0066-9] [PMID: 26286631]

[33] Thippeswamy NB, Kiran SK. Outbreak of kyasanur forest disease in shivamogga, Karnataka State, India, during 2015. SOJ Vet Sci 2017; 3(2) Available from: https://symbiosisonlinepublishing.com/veterinary-sciences/

[34] Hassall RMJ, Burthe SJ, Schäfer SM, Hartemink N, Purse BV. Using mechanistic models to highlight research priorities for tick-borne zoonotic diseases: Improving our understanding of the ecology and maintenance of Kyasanur Forest Disease in India. PLoS Negl Trop Dis 2023; 17(5): e0011300.
[http://dx.doi.org/10.1371/journal.pntd.0011300] [PMID: 37126514]

[35] Singh P, Kumar P, Dhiman RC. Kyasanur forest disease and climatic attributes in India. J Vector Borne Dis 2022; 59(1): 79-85.
[http://dx.doi.org/10.4103/0972-9062.331408] [PMID: 35708408]

[36] Soldatenko S, Bogomolov A, Ronzhin A. Mathematical modelling of climate change and variability in the context of outdoor ergonomics. Mathematics 2021; 9(22): 2920.
[http://dx.doi.org/10.3390/math9222920]

[37] Keshavamurthy R, Charles LE. Predicting Kyasanur forest disease in resource-limited settings using event-based surveillance and transfer learning. Sci Rep 2023; 13(1): 11067.
[http://dx.doi.org/10.1038/s41598-023-38074-0] [PMID: 37422454]

[38] Kasabi GS, Murhekar MV, Sandhya VK, *et al.* Coverage and effectiveness of Kyasanur forest disease (KFD) vaccine in Karnataka, South India, 2005-10. PLoS Negl Trop Dis 2013; 7(1): e2025.
[http://dx.doi.org/10.1371/journal.pntd.0002025] [PMID: 23359421]

CHAPTER 4

Climate Change and Dengue: A Growing Threat

S Binduja[1] and **Jayalakshmi Krishnan**[1,*]

[1] Vector Biology Research Laboratory, Department of Biotechnology, Central University of Tamil Nadu, Thiruvarur, India

Abstract: Climate change is a significant driver of shifts in the distribution and prevalence of vector-borne diseases, with dengue fever being a prominent example. Dengue, caused by the dengue virus and transmitted primarily by *Aedes aegypti* and *Aedes albopictus* mosquitoes, has seen a marked increase in incidence and geographic spread in recent decades. This chapter explores the multifaceted relationship between climate change and dengue transmission, highlighting how rising temperatures, altered rainfall patterns, and increased humidity contribute to mosquito proliferation and viral transmission.

Keywords: *Aedes* mosquitoes, Climate change, Deforestation, Dengue fever, Humidity, Predictive modeling, Rainfall pattern, Temperature rise, Urbanization, Vector control, Vector-borne diseases.

INTRODUCTION

Climate change refers to significant and lasting changes in temperature and weather patterns, which can be natural or due to human activities such as the burning of fossil fuels, deforestation, and industrial processes [1]. Large volumes of greenhouse gases, such as carbon dioxide and methane, are released into the atmosphere as a result of these activities, trapping heat and contributing to global warming. This phenomenon, known as global warming, is a primary driver of climate change [1]. The impacts of climate change are widespread and profound, and pose many risks to human beings and other lives on Earth [2]. Global health is particularly vulnerable, as climate change can be a reason for health problems directly and indirectly. Rising temperatures and altered weather patterns enhance heat-related illnesses and deaths. Furthermore, the distribution and activity of disease-transmitting vectors like mosquitoes can be affected by climate change, which could lead to an increase in the prevalence of vector-borne diseases [3].

* **Corresponding author Jayalakshmi Krishnan:** Vector Biology Research Laboratory, Department of Biotechnology, Central University of Tamil Nadu, Thiruvarur, India; E-mail: jayalakshmi@cutn.ac.in

Jayalakshmi Krishnan, Sigamani Panneer, P. Thiyagarajan, Balachandar Vellingiri & Pradeep Kumar Srivastava (Eds.)

Dengue fever [break-bone fever] is a viral infection spread by mosquitoes, which poses a significant public health challenge in many parts of the world [4]. It is caused by the dengue virus, which exists in four distinct serotypes [5]. The symptoms of dengue fever range from mild to severe and include high fever, severe headache, pain behind the eyes, joint and muscle pain, rash, and mild bleeding [such as nose or gum bleeding or easy bruising. One-fourth of those infected will become sick [6]. The transmission of dengue fever primarily occurs through the bite of infected female mosquitoes of the species *Aedes aegypti* and *Aedes albopictus*. These mosquitoes are highly adapted to urban environments and breed in stagnant water sources commonly found around human habitations [7]. *Aedes aegypti*, particularly, prefers biting humans, and it has the ability to survive in close proximity to human habitations [8].

In the last five years, global incidence of dengue fever has increased dramatically. Over 7.6 million dengue cases had been recorded by the WHO as of April 30, 2024, and dengue transmission is still actively observed in 90 countries, although not all cases are formally reported [9]. Many countries are endemic to dengue, including Regions of Africa, the Americas, and South East Asia. The most seriously affected areas are The Americas, South East Asia, and Western Pacific regions, with Asia accounting for about 70% of the global disease burden. In 2023, the WHO Region of the Americas reported the highest number of dengue cases, with 4.5 million cases and 2300 deaths [4]. Since 2000, the dengue outbreak has grown throughout the region, both in newly affected areas and in previously unaffected ones. The rise in dengue cases can be attributed to various factors, including increased urbanization, international travel, and, notably, climate change [10]. Warmer temperatures and altered precipitation patterns foster the growth and multiplication of *Aedes* mosquito populations, which in turn promote the spread of dengue fever to new regions and increase the frequency of outbreaks. Moreover, monsoon season provides ideal conditions for *Aedes* mosquito breeding and survival [9].

Climate change not only poses direct health risks through extreme weather events and heatwaves but also exacerbates the spread of vector-borne diseases like dengue fever. Addressing climate change and implementing effective vector control measures are crucial steps in mitigating these health impacts and protecting global populations from the escalating threat of dengue fever.

History of Dengue Fever

Some historical texts suggest that dengue-like illnesses were present as far back as 265-420 AD in China, with symptoms resembling those of modern dengue. However, the disease was not formally recognized until much later [11] [12].

18th and 19th Centuries

- **First Recorded Outbreaks:** The first documented outbreaks of dengue occurred in the Caribbean during the late 18th century. The disease spread to various parts of the Americas and was noted in Asia and Africa [13].
- **Transmission:** During this period, it became apparent that the disease was transmitted by mosquitoes, particularly *Aedes aegypti*. However, the exact mechanisms of transmission were not well understood [13].

Early 20th Century

- **Discovery of the Vector:** In the 1900s, researchers identified *Aedes* mosquitoes as the primary vectors of dengue. In 1906, the association between the mosquito and the disease was established. The first significant global epidemic of dengue fever occurred in 1950 in the Philippines, followed by outbreaks in Thailand and other Southeast Asian nations [14].

Late 20th Century to Present

- **Reemergence and Spread:** In the 1970s, dengue reemerged as a significant public health concern, particularly in tropical and subtropical regions. The disease spread to new areas, including the Americas and the Pacific Islands.
- **Dengue Hemorrhagic Fever:** In the 1980s, Dengue Hemorrhagic Fever [DHF] and Dengue Shock Syndrome [DSS] emerged as severe forms of the disease, primarily affecting children in Southeast Asia. These forms can lead to high mortality rates if not treated promptly [14].
- **Increased Incidence:** Since the 1990s, the incidence of dengue has increased dramatically, with significant outbreaks reported in Asia, Latin America, and Africa [15] [16]. The World Health Organization [WHO] has classified dengue as a major public health problem [9].

Modern Developments

- **Vaccination Efforts:** The first dengue vaccine, Dengvaxia, was approved for use in several countries in 2015. However, its efficacy is limited to individuals who have had a previous dengue infection. Research is ongoing to develop more effective vaccines [17] [18].
- **Global Response:** The WHO and various health organizations have initiated global strategies to control dengue through vector management, community education, and surveillance to mitigate outbreaks [4].

What is Dengue Fever?

Dengue fever is a mosquito-borne viral infection caused primarily by two species of mosquitoes, *Aedes aegypti* and *Aedes albopictus*. These mosquitoes are common in tropical and subtropical regions of the world, where the climate provides ideal conditions for their breeding and survival. Dengue fever is caused by one of the four closely related but antigenically distinct serotypes of the dengue virus: DENV-1, DENV-2, DENV-3, and DENV-4. Each of these serotypes belongs to the *Flavivirus* genus, which also includes viruses like Zika and Yellow Fever. As single-stranded RNA viruses, the dengue serotypes can infect humans multiple times, leading to an increased risk of severe manifestations of the disease.

When an individual is infected with one serotype of the dengue virus, they usually develop lifelong immunity against that particular serotype. However, immunity to one serotype only provides temporary cross-protection against the other three serotypes. This means that people can be infected with dengue multiple times throughout their lives, each time by a different serotype. Subsequent infections with different serotypes increase the risk of developing severe forms of the disease, such as Dengue Hemorrhagic Fever [DHF] or Dengue Shock Syndrome [DSS]. These severe manifestations are life-threatening conditions characterized by increased vascular permeability, bleeding, and potentially fatal shock. The severity of the disease is largely due to immune-mediated processes triggered by the body's response to the virus [19] [20].

The symptoms of dengue fever typically appear between 4 to 14 days after being bitten by an infected mosquito, with most cases emerging around 7 days. Common symptoms include high fever, severe headaches, pain behind the eyes, joint and muscle pain, nausea, vomiting, and the appearance of a rash. The disease is often referred to as "breakbone fever" due to the intensity of the bone and muscle pain. Symptoms usually last between 2 to 7 days, and while the disease is self-limiting in most cases, there is no specific antiviral treatment for dengue. Management largely focuses on supportive care, including fluid replacement and pain relief, with hospitalization required for severe cases of DHF and DSS [5].

Aedes mosquitoes, the primary vectors of dengue, breed in stagnant water, often found in artificial containers such as discarded tires, flower pots, buckets, and small pools of water. Urban areas, where humans and water sources are in close proximity, provide ideal breeding grounds for these mosquitoes. Unlike most other mosquito species that feed at night, *Aedes aegypti* and *Aedes albopictus* are day-biting mosquitoes, with peak feeding times occurring in the early morning and late afternoon. Female mosquitoes acquire the virus when they bite an infected person and can transmit the virus to others throughout their lifespan, spreading the disease rapidly in densely populated areas. Due to rapid urbanization and poor water management, dengue has become an increasing public health concern in many parts of the world.

Despite extensive efforts to control *Aedes* mosquito populations and limit transmission, dengue fever continues to spread globally, with millions of infections reported annually. There is currently no specific medicine or antiviral therapy to treat dengue fever, so prevention remains the key strategy for reducing its spread. Prevention methods include vector control programs aimed at reducing mosquito breeding sites, as well as personal protective measures such as using insect repellent, wearing long-sleeved clothing, and ensuring that homes are fitted with screens on windows and doors [21].

Symptoms

The initial symptoms of dengue fever typically appear 4 to 10 days after being bitten by an infected mosquito and include:

- Sudden onset of high fever [often over 104°F/40°C]
- Severe headache
- Pain behind the eyes [retro-orbital pain]
- Severe joint and muscle pain [giving it the name "breakbone fever"]
- Fatigue, nausea, and vomiting
- Skin rash, which can appear two to five days after the fever starts
- Mild bleeding, such as nose or gum bleeds, or easy bruising [22]]

In some cases, symptoms may be mild and mistaken for other viral illnesses like the flu. However, severe forms of dengue [DHF and DSS] may involve life-threatening complications, including plasma leakage, fluid accumulation, respiratory distress, severe bleeding, and organ impairment [14] [23].

Severe Dengue [DHF/DSS]

Severe dengue typically develops within 24 to 48 hours after the fever subsides. Symptoms of severe dengue include:

- Severe abdominal pain
- Persistent vomiting
- Rapid breathing
- Bleeding gums or blood in vomit or stool
- Fatigue, restlessness, and irritability. If not treated promptly, it can result in organ failure, shock, or even death [16] [24].

Diagnosis

Dengue fever is diagnosed through a combination of clinical symptoms and laboratory tests, including:

- Complete Blood Count [CBC] to check for low platelet counts and hemoconcentration
- Serological tests [IgM and IgG antibodies] to confirm recent or past infection
- NS1 antigen test to detect the virus early in the infection [25]

Treatment

There is no specific antiviral treatment for dengue fever. Management focuses on supportive care:

- Hydration therapy is critical to prevent dehydration and reduce the risk of severe complications.
- Pain relievers, such as acetaminophen, are used to alleviate pain and fever. Aspirin and Nonsteroidal Anti-inflammatory Drugs [NSAIDs] should be avoided as they can increase the risk of bleeding.
- Hospitalization may be required for severe cases, where Intravenous [IV] fluids and monitoring for complications are necessary [26].

Prevention

Preventing mosquito bites is key in controlling the spread of dengue. Some preventive measures include:

- Using insect repellents containing DEET, picaridin, or oil of lemon eucalyptus.
- Wearing long-sleeved clothing and using mosquito nets.
- Eliminating stagnant water around homes to reduce mosquito breeding sites.
- Communities are also encouraged to participate in vector control programs, which involve spraying insecticides, using larvicides in water containers, and maintaining clean environments [27] [28].

A vaccine for dengue, Dengvaxia, has been approved for use in certain countries, but it is recommended only for people who have previously been infected with the virus. It is not universally available, and vaccination programs depend on the local epidemiology of dengue [29].

The Mosquito Vector

Aedes aegypti and *Aedes albopictus* are two species of mosquitoes that are known for their transmission of highly pathogenic viruses, dengue, chikungunya, Zika and yellow fever. These mosquitoes belong to the family Culicidae [30].

Aedes aegypti

Aedes aegypti, also known as the yellow fever mosquito, is the primary vector of dengue. It is a small dark mosquito with white violin or lyre-shaped scales on the dorsal side of the thorax and has banded legs. It is predominantly an urban vector and breeds in artificial water containers, such as water storage tanks, flowerpots, and discarded tires. This species is characterized as having a strong preference for feeding on human [anthrophilic] and having a tendency to live in close association with human settlement [synanthropic] [31] [32]. It is believed that *Aedes aegypti* is native to Africa . Historical data on *Aedes aegypti's* global distribution revealed that it is nearly certain that the ancestral form of the domestic *Aedes aegypti* originated in sub-Saharan Africa. Now it has spread to many tropical and subtropical areas worldwide [16]. In Africa, *Aedes aegypti* is found in two forms: the dark-colored sylvatic *Aedes aegypti formosus* [*Aaf*] and the light-colored domestic *Aedes aegypti aegypti* [*Aaa*]. These forms interbreed, resulting in intermediate hybrids [33].

The anthropophilic form of *Aedes aegypti* relies on flooded artificial containers for its larvae and pupae habitats. Few species are known to prey on *Ae. aegypti* larvae and pupae, as most artificial containers are small, intermittently flooded, and lack predaceous aquatic insects or vertebrates. While aquatic predators like dytiscid beetles and dragonfly naiads can sometimes be found in larger containers, they are uncommon in typical *Aedes aegypti* habitats. Fish and tadpoles have been introduced into large water storage containers as a control measure for *Aedes aegypti* populations [34]. *Aedes aegypti* primarily bites during the day, being the most active two hours after sunrise and several hours before sunset, but it can also bite at night in well-lit areas. It often bites people unnoticed by approaching from behind and targeting ankles and elbows. It also bites dogs and other mammals. Only female *Aedes aegypti* bite, as they need blood to lay eggs. These mosquitoes are known for their indoor resting habits, often found in and around human dwellings [8]. *Aedes aegypti* primarily shelters and feeds inside houses, while also moving between indoor and outdoor environments. It is endophilic and endophagic, targeting human hosts for blood meals [35].

Aedes albopictus

Aedes albopictus, commonly known as the Asian tiger mosquito, is a notorious pest mosquito. It is a highly invasive species that has expanded from Southeast Asia and India to North and South America, Europe, Africa, and the Pacific. Its ability to lay desiccation-resistant eggs in natural and man-made containers has facilitated its rapid spread both within and between countries. This species has spread globally, primarily through the international trade of used tires and ornamental plants, which provide ideal breeding sites [36]. It is identifiable by its distinct black and white striped pattern on its palpus and tarsi. It shares typical morphological features with other mosquitoes in the Culicidae family, except for its pointed abdomen. Males are slightly smaller than females and have bushier antennae, while females possess a longer proboscis crucial for blood-feeding [37].

Unlike *Aedes aegypti*, *Aedes albopictus* is more adaptable to different environments, ranging from urban areas to rural and forested regions. *Aedes albopictus* displays endophilic behavior but is predominantly exophagic, biting hosts outside dwellings and feeding opportunistically on various animals, including both cold-blooded and warm-blooded species [35]. Female Asian tiger mosquitoes feed during the day with peak activity during the early morning and late afternoon. Their bites often cause itchy, red bumps on the skin but not necessarily be painful. In contrast, males do not bite and mainly consume plant nectar. This species is less anthropophilic than *Aedes aegypti* and will feed on a variety of hosts, including humans, birds, and mammals. This broader host range can influence its role in the transmission dynamics of various diseases. Asian tiger mosquitoes are active year-round in warm regions but overwinter in temperate climates. Only female mosquitoes require a blood meal to lay eggs. Female mosquitoes deposit their eggs in containers holding at least half an inch of stagnant water. This means even small objects such as a bottle cap can provide sufficient water for larval development. Breeding sites are typically near adult mosquito habitats, facilitating their life cycle and potential for disease transmission [38].

Life cycle of *Aedes* mosquitoes

Mosquitoes undergo a complex life cycle with four stages: Egg, larva [with four sub-stages], pupa, and adult (Fig. **1**). While both male and female mosquitoes feed on nectar, females also require blood from vertebrate animals to mature their eggs, typically producing 100-200 eggs per batch 3-4 days after feeding. Eggs are laid on damp surfaces within containers that hold water, turning from white to black shortly after being laid. In warm climates, eggs develop within 2-3 days, whereas in cooler climates, this process can take up to a week. They can survive in a dry state for over a year, aiding their long-distance dispersal. The hatching process of eggs varies based on temperature, humidity, and exposure to desiccation. Upon contact with water, mosquito larvae hatch and begin their development, feeding on particulate matter using specialized mouthparts. The larval phase involves growing through four instars, shedding their skins three times, and is influenced by food availability and water temperature, taking from several days to a few weeks. Males develop faster than females. The pupal stage, lasting 2-3 days depending on temperature, is the final immature phase where mosquitoes undergo transformation into adults, remaining near the water surface and not feeding. The mortality rate of pupae is very low, making their numbers a good predictor of the emerging adult population. Upon emergence, the adult mosquito rests briefly on the water surface before beginning its terrestrial phase [39].

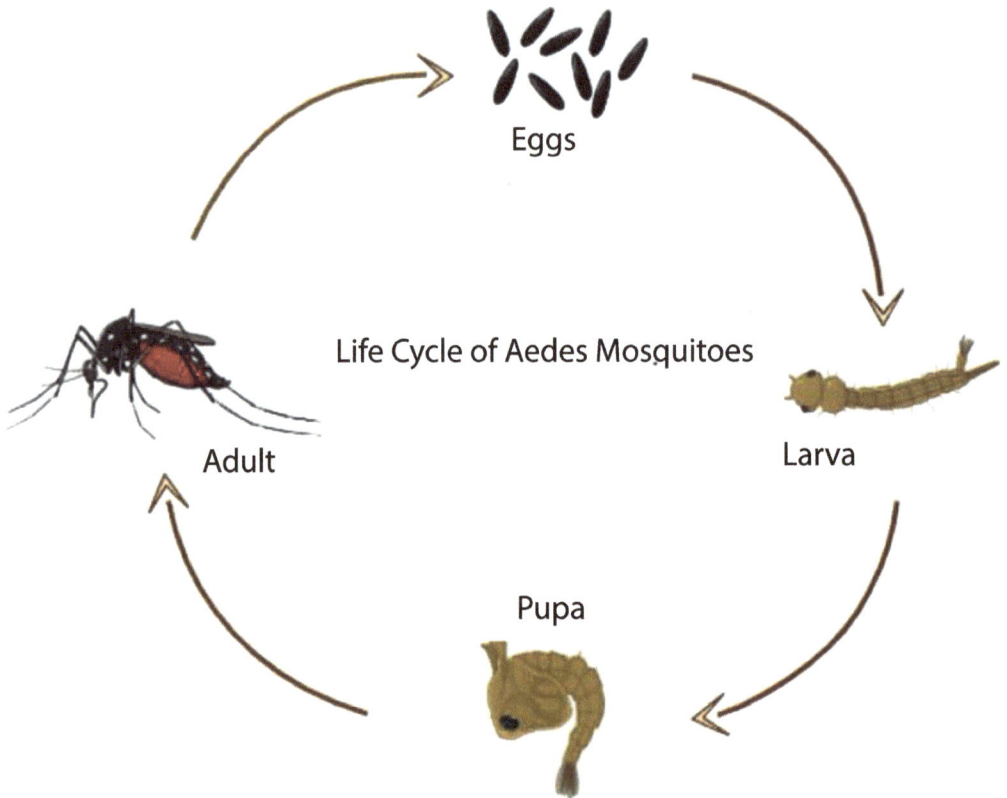

Fig. (1). Life cycle of *Aedes* mosquitoes.

Transmission of Dengue Fever

The dengue virus transmitted between human beings is through the bite of infected female *Aedes* mosquitoes [12]. Infection can be acquired through a single bite of a mosquito. Humans are the primary host, and the virus can be circulated in non-human primates and infect other mammals including pigs, marsupials, bats, birds, horses, bovids, rodents, and dogs. However, limited evidence has been found regarding dengue infection in other mammals, except bats. The mosquito becomes infected when it bites a person already infected with the dengue virus. After 4 to 10 days of incubation period, the mosquito can transmit the virus to other humans during subsequent blood meals. The virus has no adverse effect on the mosquito [40].

Several factors contribute to the spread of dengue fever:

1. **Vector Habitat**: *Aedes* mosquitoes thrive in urban and semi-urban environments. *Aedes aegypti* typically inhabit urban areas regardless of the presence of vegetation, while *Aedes albopictus* usually resides in dense arboreal vegetation. They breed in clean water containers in and around human dwellings. The habitat of *Aedes* mosquitoes is closely tied to urban environments, where they thrive in stagnant water found in containers, discarded tires, and other water-holding objects common in urban settings. Rapid urbanization, characterized by increased human population density and inadequate infrastructure, exacerbates the availability of such habitats, facilitating the breeding of *Aedes* mosquitoes. Consequently, urban areas, with their dense human populations, provide abundant blood sources for mosquitoes, enhancing the transmission cycle of dengue fever [41].
2. **Human Movement**: Travel and transportation have facilitated the spread of dengue to new areas. The human mobility from one location to another is one of the key elements contributing to the reemergence of infectious diseases. Infected individuals traveling to regions with suitable mosquito vectors can introduce the virus, initiating local transmission cycles. They assist the disease in increasing its geographic span [42].
3. **Urbanization:** The growth and population density of major cities put significant pressure on infrastructure and essential services, especially in developing countries. In response to these demands, changes in infrastructure can affect the suitability of urban areas for mosquito breeding. Irregular or absent water supply often leads to increased domestic water storage, creating more potential habitats for *Aedes aegypti*. Consequently, this can result in a more consistent and abundant supply of larval sites for these mosquitoes [34]. Rapid and unplanned urbanization, combined with climate and environmental changes, global travel, trade, and societal challenges, has stimulated the

emergence and reemergence of vector-borne diseases, particularly those transmitted by *Aedes* mosquitoes. Urbanization, characterized by increased population density and city growth, creates favorable conditions for these diseases to spread due to higher human and animal densities This process is accompanied by increased population mobility, segregation, and industrialization, impacting the dynamics of disease transmission. Effective control of *Aedes* species requires standardized measures and community-based interventions, which are challenging amid rapid urbanization [43].

4. **Climate Factors**: Dengue infections are sensitive to climate. Changes in climate factors such as temperature and rainfall influence mosquito populations and viral replication rates within mosquitoes. The temperature linked to seasonal fluctuations, is one of the most factors that influence the *Aedes* mosquito survival. Warmer temperature enhances the viral replication within the mosquito and reducing the time required for the virus to become infectious [42].

Climate Change Factors Affecting Dengue Transmission

The Earth's climate is naturally different at all times. However, its long-term state and average temperature may increase or decrease the presence of vectors. Warmer temperatures will create more suitable places for vectors to breed and survive especially in case of mosquitoes [44]. Temperature change may affect the behavior of vectors such as biting behavior of mosquitoes [45]. Extreme drought can limit the breeding and spread of mosquitoes due to water shortage. Increased rainfall can increase the amount of standing water, creating more breeding places for mosquitoes. It can happen naturally, even though human activities like deforestation, urbanization, improper waste disposal, unscientific agricultural practices, *etc.*, create more pools of standing water [46]. Change occurs as a result of a series of events that begin with the death or migration of the vector's predators and competitors, which lead to ecological release and freedom from natural restrictions [47].

Deforestation is one of the significant causes of climate change, and it has many effects on vector-borne diseases. Deforestation leads to temperature rise, cold waves, drought, severe storms, altered rain patterns, heat waves, and artificial water pools. These conditions will create geographical spread of vectors. Activities that have resulted in deforestation include agricultural activities, colonization and settlement, logging, and fuel wood collection. All these activities lead, getting more exposure to forest area, wildlife, and vectors. This increases the incidence and prevalence of diseases like dengue and other mosquito-borne diseases [48]. Deforestation and land modification promote climatic and environmental conditions that have an influence on the ecology of mosquito habitats and create new water-holding areas. Many studies are providing evidence that deforestation facilitates an increase in the transmission of vector-borne diseases as it changes the vector ecology [49]. However, depending on the ecology of vector and cycles of disease transmission, the impact of deforestation may differ for different diseases, including dengue. Few studies have investigated the relationship between dengue fever and deforestation [49]. A study conducted in Indonesia revealed dengue fever has an association with climate factors and deforestation [50]. A study from Thailand says forest area is not a risk factor for dengue fever [51]. According to a study by Christovam Barcellos, climate change and deforestation are linked to an increase in dengue fever in Brazil. The temperature has increased in some areas of Brazil due to deforestation, which triggers the transmission of dengue in those areas [52].

Temperature

Insects, as poikilotherms, are highly influenced by environmental temperature, which impacts their physiology, behavior, ecology, and ultimately, survival. They face challenges such as desiccation and metabolic changes due to daily and seasonal thermal fluctuations. Through evolutionary adaptation, insects have developed various strategies to cope with thermal stress, including heat shock protein synthesis, thermoregulation, and behavioral adjustments. Each insect species has an optimal temperature range for activities like flying and feeding, beyond which their performance declines and mortality risks increase. Factors like the physiological state and age further influence this thermal performance range, resulting in species-specific thermal niches. Some are thermal generalists, thriving across broad temperature ranges, while others are thermal specialists with narrower activity windows. These adaptations enable insects to maintain cellular integrity and optimize fitness amidst the thermal heterogeneity of their environments [35].

Temperature greatly influences the transmission of dengue virus. Temperature is closely associated with behavior and lifecycle of *Aedes* mosquitoes. Rising temperatures directly affect the survival of *Aedes* mosquitoes, biting behavior, the proliferation of dengue virus, and the vector competence to transmit dengue virus. *Aedes aegypti* and *Aedes albopictus* prefer a warm climate. Higher temperatures accelerate the mosquito life cycle, shortening the time required for the development of egg and larval phases. An increased rate of mosquito development leads to a larger mosquito population, which in turn raises the possibility of dengue transmission [53]. Biting behavior and rates of mosquitoes are highly variable and influenced by various factors including time, space, species, and climate. Moreover, temperature influences the biting behavior of mosquitoes. At lower temperatures, blood meal digestion becomes slow, lengthening the gonotrophic cycle, and reducing daily biting rates [45]. As the metabolic rates increase at higher temperatures, mosquitoes tend to bite more frequently, which enhances the dengue virus transmission potential.

Additionally, warmer temperature shortens the Extrinsic Incubation Period [EPI] of virus within the mosquito; that is, the time required for the development of the virus within mosquito before it becomes infectious [54]. The EPI is significantly reduced around 30-32°C temperatures, enabling the mosquitoes to become infectious faster than at lower temperatures. *Aedes* mosquitoes have particular temperature limits for maximum activity and survival, according to research [53].

Aedes aegypti exhibits flight activity ranging from 10°C to 35°C, with optimal sustained flight occurring between 15°C and 32°C. Flight performance peaks at 21°C, with maximum speed recorded at 32°C, suggesting adaptation for activity during cooler parts of the day and efficient flight capability across a broad temperature range [35]. There is relatively limited understanding regarding how temperature influences the flight activity and host-seeking behavior of *Aedes albopictus* [4] [35] [54]. *Aedes aegypti* typically takes multiple blood meals per gonotrophic cycle, with the frequency positively correlated with temperature. This correlation may be due to indirect effects on development and metabolic processes rather than direct impacts on blood-feeding behavior.

In contrast, *Aedes albopictus* shows variations in gonotrophic cycle duration and egg production across different constant temperatures, with optimal conditions observed around 30°C [35]. Studies on temperature fluctuations reveal that *Aedes albopictus* under varying thermal regimes can significantly impact the duration and egg-laying capacity of females. Additionally, diurnal temperature range affects *Aedes aegypti* fecundity, with broader ranges decreasing reproductive output compared to narrower temperature fluctuations. The interactions between *Aedes* mosquitoes and the dengue virus they carry are also highly sensitive to environmental conditions. Changes in temperature can affect not only mosquito development and virus replication but also mosquito-vector interactions with their human hosts. For example, at higher temperatures, mosquitoes are more active and tend to feed more frequently, increasing the probability of transmitting the virus between humans. Conversely, during colder periods, their activity is reduced, and they may become less effective vectors. However, climate change, which is leading to increased global temperatures, could expand the geographic range of *Aedes* mosquitoes, allowing them to thrive in regions that were previously too cold for them to survive. This could potentially lead to the emergence of dengue in new areas, putting previously unaffected populations at risk. Furthermore, the combination of rising temperatures and urbanization could create ideal breeding conditions for these mosquitoes, exacerbating dengue transmission in densely populated areas where mosquito-human contact is more frequent. Understanding these interactions is crucial for developing predictive models and public health strategies to manage and mitigate the impacts of dengue in a warming world [53] [54].

Rainfall Patterns

Altered rainfall patterns due to climate change also play a crucial role in dengue transmission. Rainfall has a direct impact on mosquito populations, with higher rainfall correlating to increased mosquito egg counts due to the availability of more breeding sites. Various water storage containers and discarded items that collect water during rain serve as primary breeding sites for *Aedes* mosquitoes. An abundance in the breeding sites, facilitating higher mosquito populations and, consequently, greater transmission potential. However, excessive rainfall can lead to the destruction of breeding sites and larvae, and strong winds during heavy rains can impede mosquito flight and oviposition behavior. Excessive rainfall can create more breeding habitats. It can also wash away existing larvae and eggs, temporarily reducing mosquito populations [55]. Many studies have shown that rainfall significantly influences vector distribution and dengue cases. A study from Kerala, India revealed that dengue cases rise during the monsoon season starting in June and decline post-monsoon, consistently observed over five years. Rainfall creates breeding habitats for mosquitoes, leading to their proliferation. Increased rainfall results in more breeding sites and subsequently more mosquitoes hatching. High prevalence of *Aedes aegypti* indices is reported during the monsoon and post-monsoon seasons. Wetter conditions lead to an expanded spatial range of mosquitoes and increased dengue risk [56] [46].

On the other hand, drought conditions can lead to the use of stored water by households, which can inadvertently create artificial breeding sites. In such scenarios, even small collections of water, such as those in flower pots, discarded containers, and water storage tanks, can become breeding grounds for mosquitoes. *Aedes aegypti* mosquitoes have evolved two rapidly developing genes, "tweedledee" and "tweedledum," that help them cope with drought conditions. These genes enable female mosquitoes to retain viable eggs in their ovaries for extended periods during drought conditions. This ability allows the eggs to remain viable until they can be laid in freshwater. Consequently, *Aedes aegypti* can thrive in unpredictable ecological niches with unpredictable precipitation [57]. Regions experiencing irregular rainfall patterns, with periods of intense rain followed by dry spells, may see fluctuating mosquito populations that complicate control efforts. Both excessive rainfall and drought conditions contribute to the persistence and spread of dengue, demonstrating the relationship between climate change and mosquito-borne diseases [55]. In addition to the direct effects of rainfall on mosquito breeding, the interaction between rainfall patterns and human behavior further complicates dengue transmission dynamics. During periods of heavy rain, urban areas with inadequate drainage systems often experience waterlogging, creating stagnant water bodies that serve as ideal breeding grounds for *Aedes* mosquitoes. This is particularly problematic in densely populated cities, where human exposure to mosquito bites increases due to close proximity. Moreover, after significant rainfall, people often store water in containers to prepare for potential water shortages, inadvertently creating more breeding sites [57]. Public health interventions that promote the safe storage of water and proper disposal of waste during the rainy season are therefore crucial in controlling mosquito populations. Community-level awareness campaigns that focus on eliminating standing water and cleaning potential breeding sites can reduce the risk of mosquito proliferation. Similarly, in drought-prone areas, educating communities about the risks associated with improper water storage can help mitigate the impact of mosquito breeding during dry spells. Thus, both rainfall and human responses to water availability are integral components in understanding and addressing the challenges posed by dengue in the context of climate change [56].

Humidity

The survival and development of mosquitoes are not only affected by temperature, but also by relative humidity, photoperiod, and water quality [58]. Mosquitoes require high humidity levels to maintain their water balance and avoid desiccation [34]. Studies indicate that female mosquitoes survive better and produce more eggs at moderate temperatures and higher humidity, while high temperatures and lower humidity inhibit egg-laying and reduce reproductive success [58] [59]. In tropical areas, temperatures exceeding 35 °C combined with varying humidity levels negatively impact mosquito population densities by affecting survival and reproduction [59]. While direct information on how humidity influences *Aedes albopictus* reproduction is lacking, studies show higher egg mortality for *Aedes albopictus* compared to *Aedes aegypti* at lower humidity levels, suggesting *Aedes aegypti* may better survive drier conditions [35] [58].

High humidity affects the flight activity and biting behavior of mosquitoes. In conditions of high relative humidity, mosquitoes are more active and tend to bite more frequently, thereby enhancing the transmission dynamics of dengue [60]. Conversely, low humidity can limit mosquito activity and survival, reducing the risk of dengue outbreaks [61]. However, the global trend of increasing temperatures often accompanies rising humidity levels, particularly in tropical and subtropical regions, further complicating the efforts to control mosquito populations and the spread of dengue [62].

Climate change significantly impacts *Aedes* mosquitoes and the transmission of dengue virus through alterations in temperature, humidity, and rainfall patterns. Rising temperatures accelerate mosquito life cycles, increase biting frequency, and shorten the virus's extrinsic incubation period, thereby enhancing transmission potential. Fluctuations in humidity levels affect mosquito survival, reproduction, and activity, with higher humidity promoting greater mosquito activity and biting rates, while lower humidity leads to increased egg mortality in *Aedes albopictus*. Altered rainfall patterns create more breeding sites but can also disrupt mosquito populations through excessive rainfall or drought conditions. These environmental changes underscore the complexity of controlling mosquito populations and managing dengue transmission in the face of ongoing climate change [45].

Dengue fever across the continent

Dengue fever has become the most widespread and rapidly increasing vector-borne disease globally, with 1.3 billion people at risk in Southeast Asia alone, contributing to over half of the global burden. Despite efforts, dengue cases in the region rose by 46% from 2015 to 2019, though deaths decreased slightly [63]. In 2024, Southeast Asia is experiencing a significant surge in dengue cases, notably Indonesia, with a threefold increase compared to the previous year. Bangladesh, Nepal, and Thailand have also reported higher cases, albeit with varying case fatality rates due to different reporting criteria. The surge is attributed to factors such as shifts in circulating dengue virus serotypes and favorable weather conditions during the monsoon season, which facilitate mosquito breeding. Urbanization and population movements further exacerbate the spread, increasing the risk of severe dengue and mortality across the region. These trends underscore the complex interplay of environmental, epidemiological, and socio-economic factors influencing dengue transmission in Southeast Asia [9]. The emergence of the DENV-5 serotype in Malaysia in 2007 was likely influenced by genetic changes, expansion of sylvatic cycles, and the virus's high mutation rate. Continued research is essential to comprehensively assess its epidemiology and public health implications [64]. The data shows fluctuating annual dengue cases and deaths in India, with varying peaks and declines observed across recent years. West Bengal exhibited a notable increase in cases in 2022. These trends highlight the dynamic nature of dengue transmission and the importance of ongoing surveillance and response efforts [65].

Studies reported that, as of June 2024, Latin America and the Caribbean have reported 9.3 million cases of dengue, doubling the total cases in 2023. Despite this increase, the fatality rate remains below the regional target of 0.05%. Latin American and Caribbean countries have seen significant increases in severe dengue cases and fatalities compared to 2023. The expansion of the *Aedes aegypti* mosquito's range, possibly influenced by factors like El Nino and climate change, alongside rapid urbanization and inadequate sanitation, has contributed to the spread of dengue in new areas [66] [67]. In 2024, Brazil has reported a record-breaking 5,100,766 cases of dengue fever, surpassing previous estimates [68]. Dengue outbreaks have affected 13 countries in the WHO African Region, with Burkina Faso, Mauritius, and Mali facing the highest burdens in 2024. Burkina Faso reported the majority of cases and deaths in the region, while Mauritius detected only DENV-2 serotype and Mali identified DENV-1 and DENV-3 serotypes [69].

The global burden of dengue fever continues to escalate, driven by factors such as climate change, urbanization, and viral mutations affecting transmission dynamics. Regions like Southeast Asia, Latin America, the Caribbean, and parts of Africa are experiencing unprecedented outbreaks, straining healthcare systems and underscoring the need for enhanced prevention and control measures. The emergence of new dengue virus serotypes, coupled with challenges in diagnostic capacity and vector control, further complicate efforts to mitigate the disease's impact. Continued investment in research, surveillance, and public health infrastructure is critical to managing and reducing the global burden of dengue fever effectively.

Co-infections with Other Mosquito-borne Diseases

Dengue is often found alongside other mosquito-borne diseases, particularly **chikungunya** and **Zika**, which are also transmitted by the *Aedes* mosquito. The simultaneous transmission of these diseases can lead to **co-infections**, where individuals are infected with two or more pathogens at the same time. Co-infections complicate disease diagnosis and management because the symptoms of these diseases—fever, rash, joint pain—overlap, making it difficult to distinguish one infection from another [70].

Dengue and Chikungunya: Chikungunya, characterized by severe joint pain, shares a similar transmission cycle with dengue. Both viruses often occur in the same geographical regions, making co-infection a growing concern. Patients with dengue and chikungunya co-infection experience more severe symptoms, prolonged illness, and higher morbidity compared to those infected with a single virus. These diseases share overlapping symptoms such as high fever, joint pain, headache, and rash, which complicates diagnosis and treatment. While dengue is caused by the Dengue Virus [DENV] and can lead to severe complications like dengue hemorrhagic fever or dengue shock syndrome, chikungunya, caused by the Chikungunya Virus [CHIKV], is primarily characterized by debilitating joint pain that can persist for months.

When co-infection occurs, patients often experience more severe symptoms compared to infection with just one virus. Joint pain and fever may be prolonged, leading to greater morbidity and a more challenging recovery process. This can strain healthcare systems, especially in regions where diagnostic tools to differentiate between the two diseases are limited. Co-infections of dengue and chikungunya have been reported in areas such as Southeast Asia and Latin America, where outbreaks of both viruses frequently overlap. Public health strategies focusing on vector control, early detection, and symptom management are crucial to mitigating the impact of these co-infections on affected populations [71].

Dengue and Zika: Dengue and Zika are both viral infections transmitted by *Aedes* **mosquitoes**, and co-infections with both viruses have been reported in regions like South America and Southeast Asia. Dengue, caused by the Dengue Virus [DENV], leads to high fever, muscle pain, and in severe cases, dengue hemorrhagic fever or dengue shock syndrome. Zika, caused by the Zika Virus [ZIKV], typically presents with milder symptoms such as fever, rash, and joint pain. Still, it is particularly concerning for its association with birth defects like microcephaly in pregnant women. When dengue and Zika co-infections occur, diagnosis becomes difficult due to the overlapping symptoms of fever, rash, and body aches. Co-infections can complicate clinical management and lead to more severe or prolonged symptoms, as patients deal with the immune response to both viruses simultaneously. Pregnant women are especially vulnerable, as Zika can cause serious complications for fetal development.

Efforts to control co-infections focus on vector control [eliminating mosquito breeding sites] and improving diagnostic tools to distinguish between the two viruses. Timely detection and management of co-infections are essential to minimize their health impact on affected populations. Zika virus has garnered global attention due to its association with congenital abnormalities such as microcephaly. Co-infections with dengue and Zika have been reported in regions like South America and Southeast Asia. Since both viruses are transmitted by *Aedes* mosquitoes, individuals can be exposed to both viruses in areas experiencing simultaneous outbreaks. Co-infections may increase the risk of complications, particularly in pregnant women [72] [73].

Dengue and Malaria: In some regions, particularly in sub-Saharan Africa and Southeast Asia, co-infections with dengue and malaria are a public health challenge. Regions in South Asia, Southeast Asia, and Sub-Saharan Africa often experience dengue and malaria outbreaks simultaneously, putting additional pressure on healthcare systems. Accurate diagnostic tools, along with integrated public health strategies like vector control and early detection, are crucial to managing these co-infections effectively, reducing the risk of severe disease, and improving patient recovery. While dengue is viral and malaria is parasitic, both diseases cause high fever, headache, and body aches. The dual burden of these diseases can overwhelm healthcare systems and delay appropriate treatment, leading to higher mortality rates [74]. Co-infections with dengue and malaria are challenging to diagnose due to their overlapping symptoms, particularly fever, headache, and body aches. The presence of both pathogens complicates treatment, as dengue primarily requires supportive care, while malaria necessitates specific antimalarial medications. Misdiagnosis or delayed diagnosis in co-infection cases can lead to improper treatment, worsening patient outcomes [75].

Health Implications and Challenges

Co-infections create significant challenges in clinical settings. Symptoms like fever, muscle pain, joint pain, and rashes are common to many mosquito-borne diseases, complicating diagnosis. A lack of diagnostic tools capable of differentiating between these infections further hampers effective treatment. For instance, while dengue requires supportive care, diseases like malaria may need specific antimalarial treatments. Misdiagnosis can lead to improper management, potentially worsening patient outcomes.

Furthermore, the presence of multiple infections can exacerbate the immune response, leading to more severe manifestations of illness. For example, studies have suggested that co-infection with dengue and chikungunya can result in prolonged fever and increased joint pain, making the disease more debilitating. In some cases, co-infections may even increase the risk of fatal outcomes, particularly if healthcare systems are overwhelmed or lacking in resources [76].

Prevention and Control Measures

Addressing the dual threat of dengue and co-infections requires an integrated approach to **vector control**, **public health education**, and **early diagnosis**. Effective mosquito control measures, such as **reducing breeding sites**, **using insecticides**, and **promoting personal protective behaviors** [like using bed nets and repellents], are essential in controlling the spread of these diseases. Additionally, improving diagnostic capacities to detect co-infections early can lead to better clinical outcomes.

Vaccination efforts are also advancing. Although the dengue vaccine **Dengvaxia** is available, its use is limited to individuals with previous dengue exposure due to concerns over severe disease in dengue-naïve individuals. Research into vaccines for chikungunya and Zika is ongoing, and the development of multi-target vaccines could potentially reduce the burden of co-infections in the future [77].

As the global climate continues to change, the burden of dengue and co-infections is likely to grow, particularly in regions already prone to mosquito-borne diseases. The increased spread of mosquitoes, coupled with overlapping outbreaks of diseases like Zika and chikungunya, calls for a coordinated global response. Public health systems must be equipped to handle the diagnostic challenges of co-infections, and effective vector control and preventive measures should be scaled up to mitigate the impact of these diseases on vulnerable populations.

Predictive Models and Future Projections

Integration of Climate Data

Climate models incorporate data on temperature and precipitation patterns, which are crucial for understanding mosquito population dynamics and dengue transmission. These models use historical climate data and future climate projections to predict changes in these variables. Models also consider humidity levels and the frequency and intensity of extreme weather events like floods and droughts, which can impact mosquito breeding and survival. Scientists use climate models to create different scenarios based on varying levels of greenhouse gas emissions and climate change mitigation efforts. These scenarios help predict how dengue transmission might change under different climate futures. Predictive models are essential tools for understanding the potential future trajectories of dengue transmission, particularly in the context of climate change. These models integrate various types of environmental, biological, and social data to forecast how changing conditions might affect the spread of dengue [78]. A key element in these models is the inclusion of climate data, which helps researchers better understand the intricate relationship between environmental conditions and mosquito population dynamics, as well as dengue transmission patterns. One of the most significant climatic factors influencing mosquito populations is temperature. *Aedes* mosquitoes, the primary vectors for dengue, are highly sensitive to temperature variations. Warmer temperatures can shorten the mosquito life cycle, accelerate the virus replication rate inside the mosquito, and extend the breeding season, leading to larger and more persistent mosquito populations. Predictive models use historical temperature data to assess past patterns and apply future climate projections to forecast how rising global temperatures might affect mosquito abundance and disease transmission. Increased temperatures in tropical and subtropical regions, where dengue is already endemic, are likely to intensify the disease's spread, while warming trends in temperate regions could expand the geographic range of dengue transmission into areas that have historically been free of the virus [79].

Precipitation patterns are another critical factor integrated into climate models. Rainfall influences the availability of standing water, which is essential for mosquito breeding. Predictive models take into account historical rainfall data as well as future projections to estimate changes in mosquito breeding habitats. Increased rainfall, particularly in urban areas with poor drainage systems, can lead to an abundance of water-filled containers, such as discarded tires and buckets, creating ideal conditions for *Aedes* mosquitoes to thrive. On the other hand, climate models also consider the effects of droughts, which may reduce available breeding sites in some regions but can lead to an increase in mosquito breeding in stored water containers, thus sustaining dengue transmission [80]. By modeling different rainfall patterns under various climate scenarios, scientists can better anticipate the areas and seasons most at risk of intensified dengue outbreaks. Humidity levels, often overlooked in basic models, play a significant role in mosquito survival and the transmission potential of the dengue virus. Higher humidity improves mosquito survival rates and extends their lifespan, giving them more time to transmit the virus. Climate models account for changes in humidity, particularly in regions experiencing significant fluctuations due to climate change, to refine predictions of how conducive the environment will be for mosquito populations in the future. Extreme weather events, such as floods and droughts, are becoming more frequent and intense due to climate change. Flooding can create vast breeding grounds for mosquitoes, while droughts may lead to increased reliance on water storage systems, inadvertently providing breeding habitats for mosquitoes. Predictive models incorporate these events to understand their short- and long-term effects on mosquito populations and dengue transmission. For instance, after a flood, the immediate surge in water levels can create numerous temporary mosquito habitats, leading to a spike in transmission. By analyzing the potential frequency and severity of such events under different climate scenarios, researchers can predict periods of heightened dengue risk [81].

Scientists utilize climate models to generate different scenarios based on varying levels of greenhouse gas emissions and climate change mitigation efforts. These scenarios range from high-emission, worst-case scenarios with minimal mitigation to more optimistic scenarios that assume substantial efforts to reduce emissions and limit global temperature increases. By examining multiple scenarios, predictive models offer a comprehensive view of the future risk landscape for dengue. For example, in a scenario with high greenhouse gas emissions, rising temperatures and more extreme weather events may lead to a dramatic expansion of dengue transmission zones. Conversely, under a scenario with significant climate mitigation efforts, temperature increases may be limited, and the spread of dengue may be curtailed. Incorporating climate data into predictive models allows scientists to forecast future dengue trends more accurately and provides crucial insights for public health planning. These models can help governments and health organizations prepare for future outbreaks by identifying high-risk areas, guiding mosquito control efforts, and informing vaccine distribution strategies. Additionally, predictive models serve as a valuable tool for raising awareness about the interconnectedness of climate change and infectious diseases, emphasizing the need for coordinated global efforts to reduce emissions and adapt to the health challenges posed by a warming world [82].

Epidemiological Models

Epidemiological models are vital tools in understanding and forecasting the spread of infectious diseases like dengue fever. These models help scientists estimate important metrics, such as the basic Reproduction Number [R_0], which measures the transmissibility of a disease. R_0 represents the average number of secondary infections generated by one infected individual in a fully susceptible population. In the context of dengue, R_0 is influenced by several factors, including climate variables, vector [mosquito] capacity, and human behavior. By analyzing these factors, scientists can assess the potential for dengue outbreaks and determine the conditions that might lead to sustained transmission. Climate variables, particularly temperature and precipitation, play a critical role in influencing R_0. Warmer temperatures can accelerate the development of *Aedes* mosquitoes, shorten their breeding cycles, and increase the efficiency of dengue virus replication within the mosquito, ultimately leading to a higher R_0. In contrast, cooler temperatures can slow down these processes and reduce transmission. Precipitation patterns are equally important because rain provides breeding sites for mosquitoes, which, in turn, affects mosquito population density. By including these variables in epidemiological models, scientists can estimate how R_0 will change under different climate scenarios, helping predict future dengue transmission patterns [83] [84].

In addition to climate factors, vector capacity is another important consideration in determining R_0. Vector capacity refers to the ability of *Aedes* mosquitoes to transmit the dengue virus. This is influenced by several factors, such as mosquito lifespan, biting frequency, and the mosquito's likelihood of becoming infected after biting an infected human. Changes in mosquito population density, driven by environmental factors like urbanization, deforestation, or the availability of breeding sites, also influence vector capacity. Epidemiological models take these factors into account to provide a more comprehensive understanding of how mosquito behavior affects dengue transmission. Human behavior is another key component in epidemiological models. Human movement, urbanization patterns, and efforts to control mosquito populations [such as the use of insecticides or removal of breeding sites] can all affect dengue transmission dynamics. For instance, densely populated urban areas with poor sanitation and water storage practices can increase the risk of dengue outbreaks, as they create ideal conditions for mosquito breeding. Similarly, changes in human mobility—whether due to migration, travel, or seasonal labor—can introduce the virus to new regions or intensify transmission in areas where dengue is already present. Incorporating these behavioral aspects allows scientists to model how human factors influence the spread of dengue and its R_0 in different settings. Agent-Based Models [ABMs] are another sophisticated tool used to simulate the complex interactions between mosquitoes, humans, and the environment at an individual level. Unlike traditional epidemiological models, which often use aggregate data, ABMs simulate the behavior and interactions of individual agents [in this case, mosquitoes and humans] within a virtual environment. These models can incorporate detailed climate data, such as temperature and rainfall patterns, to predict how environmental changes will influence mosquito behavior, breeding, and transmission of the dengue virus. ABMs are especially useful in capturing the fine-scale dynamics of dengue transmission, such as how changes in local temperature might alter mosquito biting patterns or how human movement can influence the spread of the virus within a specific community [85].

By combining epidemiological models with climate projections and detailed environmental data, scientists can create risk maps that highlight areas at the highest risk of dengue transmission. These maps take into account factors like temperature, precipitation, mosquito density, and human population density to forecast where future outbreaks are most likely to occur. For instance, risk maps might identify regions that are currently dengue-free but are projected to become suitable for transmission due to rising temperatures or changes in precipitation patterns. These maps are invaluable tools for public health planning, as they help governments and health organizations allocate resources efficiently, target mosquito control efforts, and plan for future vaccination campaigns. Epidemiological models, particularly those that integrate climate data, are also instrumental in guiding policy decisions. For example, these models can be used to assess the impact of different interventions, such as insecticide spraying, public education campaigns, or vaccination programs, on reducing R_0 and preventing dengue outbreaks. Policymakers can use the insights from these models to prioritize interventions that will have the greatest impact in high-risk areas, ensuring that resources are deployed where they are most needed [86].

Vector-Borne Disease Models

Vector-borne disease models are crucial for understanding and predicting the transmission dynamics of dengue fever, especially as climate change alters the environmental conditions that influence mosquito populations. One key type of model used in this field is dynamic models, which simulate the entire transmission cycle of dengue. These models account for the life stages of *Aedes* mosquitoes, from egg to larva to adult, as well as the incubation period of the dengue virus within the mosquito. Additionally, they simulate the virus's transmission to humans when a mosquito bites an infected person and subsequently spreads the virus to others. Climate data plays a pivotal role in dynamic models, as it adjusts key parameters such as mosquito lifespan, breeding rates, and biting frequency. For instance, warmer temperatures can accelerate mosquito development and viral replication within the mosquito, while variations in rainfall can affect the availability of breeding sites. By integrating these factors, dynamic models can predict how changes in temperature, humidity, and precipitation will influence the overall transmission dynamics of dengue. Spatial models, on the other hand, use Geographic Information Systems [GIS] to map the distribution of dengue cases and predict where future outbreaks are likely to occur. These models incorporate environmental and climate data, such as temperature trends, precipitation patterns, and human population density, to identify geographic regions at higher risk of dengue outbreaks. With the use of GIS technology, spatial models can provide detailed, location-specific risk maps that help public health officials and governments plan targeted interventions, such as mosquito control measures and vaccination campaigns, in areas most vulnerable to dengue outbreaks [87].

By combining both dynamic and spatial models, scientists can create robust predictive frameworks that offer insights into how dengue might spread under different climate scenarios. These models are particularly valuable for public health planning, as they help identify future hotspots and enable timely interventions to protect vulnerable populations. In the context of a warming planet, these models are indispensable for guiding strategies to mitigate the growing threat of dengue, ensuring resources are allocated efficiently and that high-risk regions are prioritized for preventive measures [88].

Mathematical Model

Mathematical models for dengue provide a structured framework to analyze the complex dynamics of vector-borne diseases, capturing the interactions between hosts, vectors, and environmental factors that drive changes in disease epidemiology. The Susceptible-Exposed-Infectious-Recovered [SEIR] model for dengue fever divides the human population into four compartments: Susceptible,

Exposed, Infectious, and Recovered, and the mosquito population into Susceptible, Exposed, and Infectious. It uses differential equations to describe how individuals move between compartments based on transmission rates, incubation periods, and recovery rates. The model captures the interaction between humans and mosquitoes, where mosquitoes become infected by biting an infectious human and later transmit the virus to susceptible humans after an extrinsic incubation period. Environmental factors, such as temperature and rainfall, influence key parameters like mosquito survival and virus replication rates. This model helps predict dengue outbreaks, evaluate control strategies, and assess the impact of climate change on disease dynamics [89].

The vectorial capacity model quantifies the potential of mosquito populations to transmit diseases like dengue. It integrates factors such as mosquito density, biting frequency, survival rates, and the extrinsic incubation period of the pathogen within the vector. By analyzing these parameters, the model estimates the rate at which new infections occur from an existing case, aiding in understanding and predicting disease transmission dynamics [90]. The Ross-Macdonald model for dengue provides insights into the magnitude and recurrence of outbreaks by incorporating factors such as human movement and mosquito seasonal variations. The model highlights the role of human mobility and localized environmental conditions in shaping the frequency and scale of dengue outbreaks [91]. The agent-based model for dengue simulates interactions between humans and mosquitoes in a spatiotemporal environment, extending the traditional SEIR framework. It incorporates mosquito density and behavior to predict virus transmission and spread in specific areas, offering visualization and forecasting capabilities [85]. Mathematical models offer valuable insights into the dynamics of disease transmission by analyzing human-vector interactions, environmental factors, and intervention impacts. These models are essential for predicting outbreaks, optimizing control strategies, and understanding the influence of climate change on the epidemiology of dengue.

Mitigation and Adaptation Strategies

Mitigation and adaptation strategies to address the impact of climate change on dengue fever encompass public health interventions, policy measures, and technological innovations. Public health interventions focus on mosquito control programs, vaccination efforts, and community education. Effective mosquito control includes managing larval sources, using insecticides, and employing biological and genetic control methods [92]. Vaccination efforts involve developing and distributing vaccines, such as Dengvaxia, and implementing immunization programs in endemic areas [93]. Community education emphasizes public awareness campaigns, community participation, and school programs to teach preventive measures.

Policy measures are crucial for a coordinated response to climate-driven health risks. National policies include adopting Integrated Vector Management [IVM], strengthening health systems, and establishing climate-health surveillance systems [92]. International policies involve global health initiatives led by organizations like WHO and PAHO, securing funding and technical support for dengue control, and integrating health considerations into international climate agreements [93]. These policies ensure a comprehensive and unified approach to managing the health impacts of climate change.

Technological innovations play a significant role in enhancing dengue surveillance and vector control. Advanced surveillance tools, such as remote sensing and GIS, help monitor mosquito habitats and predict outbreaks, while mobile apps facilitate real-time data collection [94]. New vector control technologies include developing innovative insecticides, introducing Wolbachia-infected mosquitoes to reduce dengue transmission, and using the Sterile Insect Technique [SIT] to lower mosquito populations [95]. Additionally, building climate-resilient healthcare facilities and implementing early warning systems based on climate data are vital for effective dengue prevention and response. Integrating these strategies enhances community resilience and mitigates the adverse effects of climate change on dengue fever.

CONCLUSION

The intersection of climate change and dengue fever presents a formidable challenge that requires a coordinated global response. The evidence is clear: rising temperatures, altered rainfall patterns, and increasing humidity directly influence the lifecycle, behavior, and distribution of *Aedes* mosquitoes, thereby amplifying the risk of dengue transmission. Deforestation, urbanization, and other human activities exacerbate these climate effects, creating more breeding sites and increasing human exposure to mosquito vectors.

REFERENCES

[1]   Nations U. United Nations. United Nations. 2024. What Is Climate Change? Available from: https://www.un.org/en/climatechange/what-is-climate-change

[2]   Nations U. United Nations. United Nations. 2024. Causes and Effects of Climate Change. Available from: https://www.un.org/en/climatechange/science/causes-effects-climate-change

[3]   WHO. Climate change. 2023. Available from: https://www.who.int/news-room/fac-sheets/detail/climate-change-and-health

[4]   W.H.O. Dengue and severe dengue. 2024. Available from: https://www.who.int/news-room/fac-sheets/detail/dengue-and-severe-dengue

[5]   CDC. Dengue. 2024. About Dengue. Available from: https://www.cdc.gov/dengue/about/index.html

[6]   CDC. Dengue. 2024. Symptoms of Dengue and Testing. Available from: https://www.cdc.gov/dengue/signs-symptoms/index.html

[7]   Islam MT, Quispe C, Herrera-Bravo J, *et al.* Production, transmission, pathogenesis, and control of dengue virus: A literature-based undivided perspective. BioMed Res Int 2021; 2021(1): 4224816.
[http://dx.doi.org/10.1155/2021/4224816] [PMID: 34957305]

[8]   Seda H. Dengue and the Aedes aegypti mosquito

[9]   W.H.O. Dengue - Global situation. 2024. Available from: https://www.who.int/emergencies/disease-outbreak-news/item/2024-DON518

[10] Epidemiology, burden of disease and transmission. Dengue: guidelines for diagnosis, treatment, prevention and control: new edition 2009. Available from: https://www.ncbi.nlm.nih.gov/books/NBK143159/

[11] Murray NEA, Quam MB, Wilder-Smith A. Epidemiology of dengue: past, present and future prospects. Clin Epidemiol 2013; 5: 299-309.
[PMID: 23990732]

[12] Ooi EE. The re-emergence of dengue in China. BMC Med 2015; 13(1): 99.
[http://dx.doi.org/10.1186/s12916-015-0345-0] [PMID: 25925732]

[13] Gubler DJ. Dengue and dengue hemorrhagic fever. Clin Microbiol Rev 1998; 11(3): 480-96.
[http://dx.doi.org/10.1128/CMR.11.3.480] [PMID: 9665979]

[14] Kuno G. Emergence of the severe syndrome and mortality associated with dengue and dengue-like illness: historical records (1890 to 1950) and their compatibility with current hypotheses on the shift of disease manifestation. Clin Microbiol Rev 2009; 22(2): 186-201.
[http://dx.doi.org/10.1128/CMR.00052-08] [PMID: 19366911]

[15] Ilic I, Ilic M. Global patterns of trends in incidence and mortality of dengue, 1990–2019: An analysis based on the global burden of disease study. Medicina (Kaunas) 2024; 60(3): 425.
[http://dx.doi.org/10.3390/medicina60030425] [PMID: 38541151]

[16] Zeng Z, Zhan J, Chen L, Chen H, Cheng S. Global, regional, and national dengue burden from 1990 to 2017: A systematic analysis based on the global burden of disease study 2017. EClinicalMedicine 2021; 32: 100712.
[http://dx.doi.org/10.1016/j.eclinm.2020.100712] [PMID: 33681736]

[17] Foucambert P, Esbrand FD, Zafar S, *et al.* Efficacy of dengue vaccines in the prevention of severe dengue in children: A systematic review. Cureus 2022; 14(9): e28916.
[http://dx.doi.org/10.7759/cureus.28916] [PMID: 36225478]

[18] Vaccines and immunization: Dengue. 2024. Available from: https://www.who.int/news-room/questions-and-answers/item/dengue-vaccines

[19] Schaefer TJ, Panda PK, Wolford RW. Dengue Fever. In: StatPearls. Treasure Island: StatPearls Publishing, 2024. Available from: http://www.ncbi.nlm.nih.gov/books/NBK430732/

[20] Cattarino L, Rodriguez-Barraquer I, Imai N, Cummings DAT, Ferguson NM. Mapping global variation in dengue transmission intensity. Sci Transl Med 2020; 12(528): eaax4144.
[http://dx.doi.org/10.1126/scitranslmed.aax4144] [PMID: 31996463]

[21] McNaughton D, Miller ER, Tsourtos G. The importance of water typologies in lay entomologies of *Aedes aegypti* habitat, breeding and dengue risk: A study from Northern Australia. Trop Med Infect Dis 2018; 3(2): 67.
[http://dx.doi.org/10.3390/tropicalmed3020067] [PMID: 30274463]

[22] Khosavanna RR, Kareko BW, Brady AC, *et al.* Clinical symptoms of dengue infection among patients from a non-endemic area and potential for a predictive model: A multiple logistic regression analysis

and decision tree. Am J Trop Med Hyg 2021; 104(1): 121-9.
[http://dx.doi.org/10.4269/ajtmh.20-0192] [PMID: 33200724]

[23]   Umakanth M, Suganthan N. Unusual manifestations of dengue fever: A review on expanded dengue syndrome. Cureus 2020; 12(9): e10678.
[http://dx.doi.org/10.7759/cureus.10678] [PMID: 33133844]

[24]   Weltgesundheitsorganisation, editor Dengue haemorrhagic fever: diagnosis, treatment, prevention and control 2. ed.. 1997; 1-84.

[25]   Laboratory diagnosis and diagnostic tests. Dengue: guidelines for diagnosis, treatment, prevention and control: new edition 2009. Available from: https://www.ncbi.nlm.nih.gov/books/NBK143156/

[26]   Gan VC. Dengue: Moving from current standard of care to state-of-the-art treatment. Curr Treat Options Infect Dis 2014; 6(3): 208-26.
[http://dx.doi.org/10.1007/s40506-014-0025-1] [PMID: 25999799]

[27]   Tayal A, Kabra SK, Lodha R. Management of dengue: An updated review. Indian J Pediatr 2023; 90(2): 168-77.
[http://dx.doi.org/10.1007/s12098-022-04394-8] [PMID: 36574088]

[28]   CDC.   Dengue.   2024.   Preventing   Dengue.   Available   from:
https://www.cdc.gov/dengue/prevention/index.html

[29]   W.H.O. Vaccines and immunization: Dengue. 2024. Available from: https://www.who.int/news-room/questions-and-answers/item/dengue-vaccines

[30]   Ahebwa A, Hii J, Neoh KB, Chareonviriyaphap T. *Aedes aegypti* and *Aedes albopictus* (Diptera: Culicidae) ecology, biology, behaviour, and implications on arbovirus transmission in Thailand: Review. One Health 2023; 16: 100555.
[http://dx.doi.org/10.1016/j.onehlt.2023.100555] [PMID: 37363263]

[31]   Madariaga M, Ticona E, Resurreccion C. Chikungunya: bending over the Americas and the rest of the world. Braz J Infect Dis 2015; 20
[http://dx.doi.org/DOI: 10.1016/j.bjid.2015.10.004] [PMID: 26707971]

[32]   *Aedes   aegypti* -   an   overview | ScienceDirect   Topics.   2024.   Available   from:
https://www.sciencedirect.com/topics/immunology-and-microbiology/aedes-aegypti

[33]   Powell JR, Tabachnick WJ. History of domestication and spread of *Aedes aegypti* - A Review. Mem Inst Oswaldo Cruz 2013; 108(Suppl 1) (Suppl. 1): 11-7.
[http://dx.doi.org/10.1590/0074-0276130395] [PMID: 24473798]

[34]   Egid BR, Coulibaly M, Dadzie SK, *et al.* Review of the ecology and behaviour of *Aedes aegypti* and *Aedes albopictus* in Western Africa and implications for vector control. Current Research in Parasitology & Vector-Borne Diseases 2022; 2: 100074.
[http://dx.doi.org/10.1016/j.crpvbd.2021.100074] [PMID: 35726222]

[35]   OECD. Ecology of the mosquito *Ae. aegypti*. Safety Assess Transgenic Organisms Environ. Paris 2018; pp. 91-105.
[http://dx.doi.org/10.1787/9789264302235-8-en]

[36]   Reinhold J, Lazzari C, Lahondère C. Effects of the environmental temperature on *Aedes aegypti* and *Aedes albopictus* mosquitoes: A review. Insects 2018; 9(4): 158.
[http://dx.doi.org/10.3390/insects9040158] [PMID: 30404142]

[37]   van den Hurk AF, Nicholson J, Beebe NW, *et al.* Ten years of the Tiger: *Aedes albopictus* presence in Australia since its discovery in the Torres Strait in 2005. One Health 2016; 2: 19-24.
[http://dx.doi.org/10.1016/j.onehlt.2016.02.001] [PMID: 28616473]

[38]   James E. Maruniak LR. Asian tiger mosquito - *Aedes albopictus* [Skuse]. 2024. Available from: https://entnemdept.ufl.edu/creatures/aquatic/asian_tiger.htm

[39]   National Pest Management Association. Asian Tiger Mosquitoes Facts & Info: Tiger Mosquito Bites.

2024. Available from: https://www.pestworld.org/pest-guide/mosquitoes/asian-tiger-mosquitoes/

[40]   Chouin-Carneiro T, Santos FB dos, Chouin-Carneiro T, Santos FB dos. Transmission of major arboviruses in Brazil: the role of *Aedes aegypti* and *Aedes albopictus* vectors. Biol Control Pest Vector Insects 2017. Available from: https://www.intechopen.com/chapters/53702

[41]   Gwee SXW, St John AL, Gray GC, Pang J. Animals as potential reservoirs for dengue transmission: A systematic review. One Health 2021; 12: 100216.
[http://dx.doi.org/10.1016/j.onehlt.2021.100216] [PMID: 33598525]

[42]   Global Vector Hub. The *Aedes* Mosquito Global Vector Hub. 2009 Available from: https://globalvectorhub.tghn.org/vector-species/aedes-mosquito/

[43]   Phaijoo GR, Gurung DB. Modeling impact of temperature and human movement on the persistence of dengue disease. Comput Math Methods Med 2017; 2017: 1-9.
[http://dx.doi.org/10.1155/2017/1747134] [PMID: 29312458]

[44]   Kolimenakis A, Heinz S, Wilson ML, *et al.* The role of urbanisation in the spread of *Aedes* mosquitoes and the diseases they transmit—A systematic review. PLoS Negl Trop Dis 2021; 15(9): e0009631.
[http://dx.doi.org/10.1371/journal.pntd.0009631] [PMID: 34499653]

[45]   Mojahed N, Mohammadkhani MA, Mohamadkhani A. Climate crises and developing vector-borne diseases: A narrative review. Iran J Public Health 2022; 51(12): 2664-73.
[http://dx.doi.org/10.18502/ijph.v51i12.11457] [PMID: 36742229]

[46]   Zahid MH, Van Wyk H, Morrison AC, *et al.* The biting rate of *Aedes aegypti* and its variability: A systematic review (1970–2022). PLoS Negl Trop Dis 2023; 17(8): e0010831.
[http://dx.doi.org/10.1371/journal.pntd.0010831] [PMID: 37552669]

[47]   Madi M, Ahmad R, Mohd Kulaimi N, Ali W, Ismail S, Lim LH. Climatic influences on *Aedes* mosquito larvae population. Malays J Sci 2012; 31: 30-9.

[48]   Moore SM, Borer ET, Hosseini PR. Predators indirectly control vector-borne disease: linking predator–prey and host–pathogen models. J R Soc Interface 2010; 7(42): 161-76.
[http://dx.doi.org/10.1098/rsif.2009.0131] [PMID: 19474078]

[49]   Karuppusamy B, Sarma DK, Lalmalsawma P, Pautu L, Karmodiya K, Balabaskaran Nina P. Effect of climate change and deforestation on vector borne diseases in the North-Eastern Indian State of Mizoram bordering Myanmar. Journal of Climate Change and Health 2021; 2: 100015.
[http://dx.doi.org/10.1016/j.joclim.2021.100015]

[50]   Kalbus A, de Souza Sampaio V, Boenecke J, Reintjes R. Exploring the influence of deforestation on dengue fever incidence in the Brazilian Amazonas state. PLoS One 2021; 16(1): e0242685.
[http://dx.doi.org/10.1371/journal.pone.0242685] [PMID: 33411795]

[51]   Husnina Z, Clements ACA, Wangdi K. Forest cover and climate as potential drivers for dengue fever in Sumatra and Kalimantan 2006–2016: a spatiotemporal analysis. Trop Med Int Health 2019; 24(7): 888-98.
[http://dx.doi.org/10.1111/tmi.13248] [PMID: 31081162]

[52]   Nakhapakorn K, Tripathi N. An information value based analysis of physical and climatic factors affecting dengue fever and dengue haemorrhagic fever incidence. Int J Health Geogr 2005; 4(1): 13.
[http://dx.doi.org/10.1186/1476-072X-4-13] [PMID: 15943863]

[53]   Fiocruz. Fiocruz. Increase in dengue cases is linked to climate change and deforestation in Brazil. 2024. Available from: https://portal.fiocruz.br/en/news/2024/03/increase-dengue-cases-linked-climate-change-and-deforestation-brazil

[54]   Liu Z, Zhang Q, Li L, *et al.* The effect of temperature on dengue virus transmission by *Aedes* mosquitoes. Front Cell Infect Microbiol 2023; 13: 1242173.
[http://dx.doi.org/10.3389/fcimb.2023.1242173] [PMID: 37808907]

[55]   Kamiya T, Greischar MA, Wadhawan K, Gilbert B, Paaijmans K, Mideo N. Temperature-dependent

variation in the extrinsic incubation period elevates the risk of vector-borne disease emergence. Epidemics 2020; 30: 100382.
[http://dx.doi.org/10.1016/j.epidem.2019.100382] [PMID: 32004794]

[56]   Gopalsamy B, Yazan LS, Razak NNA, Man M. Association of temperature and rainfall with *Aedes* mosquito population in 17th College of Universiti Putra Malaysia. 2021.

[57]   Nair DG, Aravind NP. Association between rainfall and the prevalence of clinical cases of dengue in Thiruvananthapuram district, India. Int J Mosq Res 2020; 7(6): 46-50.
[http://dx.doi.org/10.22271/23487941.2020.v7.i6a.488]

[58]   Venkataraman K, Shai N, Lakhiani P, Zylka S, Zhao J, Herre M, *et al.* Rapidly evolving genes underlie *Aedes aegypti* mosquito reproductive resilience during drought. 2022.
[http://dx.doi.org/10.1101/2022.03.01.482582]

[59]   Cai X, Zhao J, Deng H, *et al.* Effects of temperature, relative humidity, and illumination on the entomological parameters of *Aedes albopictus*: an experimental study. Int J Biometeorol 2023; 67(4): 687-94.
[http://dx.doi.org/10.1007/s00484-023-02446-y] [PMID: 36884085]

[60]   Costa EAPA, Santos EMM, Correia JC, Albuquerque CMR. Impact of small variations in temperature and humidity on the reproductive activity and survival of *Aedes aegypti* (Diptera, Culicidae). Rev Bras Entomol 2010; 54(3): 488-93. [Diptera, Culicidae].
[http://dx.doi.org/10.1590/S0085-56262010000300021]

[61]   Rueda LM, Patel KJ, Axtell RC, Stinner RE. Temperature-dependent development and survival rates of *Culex quinquefasciatus* and *Aedes aegypti* (Diptera: Culicidae). J Med Entomol 1990; 27(5): 892-8.
[http://dx.doi.org/10.1093/jmedent/27.5.892] [PMID: 2231624]

[62]   Reiter P. Weather, Vector Biology, and Arboviral Recrudescence. The Arboviruses. Epidemiology and Ecology 2020; pp. 245-56.

[63]   Hales S, de Wet N, Maindonald J, Woodward A. Potential effect of population and climate changes on global distribution of dengue fever: an empirical model. Lancet 2002; 360(9336): 830-4.
[http://dx.doi.org/10.1016/S0140-6736(02)09964-6] [PMID: 12243917]

[64]   W.H.O. Dengue in South-East Asia. 2024. Available from: https://www.who.int/southeastasia/health-topics/dengue-and-severe-dengue

[65]   Mustafa MS, Rasotgi V, Jain S, Gupta V. Discovery of fifth serotype of dengue virus (DENV-5): A new public health dilemma in dengue control. Med J Armed Forces India 2015; 71(1): 67-70.
[http://dx.doi.org/10.1016/j.mjafi.2014.09.011] [PMID: 25609867]

[66]   NCVBDC. Dengue situation in india. National Center for Vector Borne Diseases Control [NCVBDC]. 2024. Available from: https://ncvbdc.mohfw.gov.in/index4.php?lang=1&level=0&linkid=431&lid=3715

[67]   PAHO. Despite record dengue cases, Latin America and the Caribbean maintain a low fatality rate - PAHO/WHO | Pan American Health Organization. 2024. Available from: https://www.paho.org/en/news/20-6-2024-despite-record-dengue-case--latin-america-and-caribbean-maintain-low-fatality-rate

[68]   Carlos G Torres V JRTR. Dengue in Latin America – a unique situation. Dengue Bull 2002; 26 Available from: https://iris.who.int/bitstream/handle/10665/163727/dbv26p62.pdf;sequence=1

[69]   Lacerda Nara. Brazil surpasses 5 million cases of dengue. Brasil de Fato 2024. Available from: https://www.brasildefato.com.br/2024/05/21/brazil-surpasses-5-million-cases-of-dengue

[70]   Turuk J, Palo SK, Rath S, *et al.* Viral characteristics and clinical presentation in dengue co-infection-Findings from a facility based observational study in Odisha, India. J Family Med Prim Care 2021; 10(8): 2958-63.
[http://dx.doi.org/10.4103/jfmpc.jfmpc_2380_20] [PMID: 34660431]

[71]   Rezza G. Dengue and chikungunya: long-distance spread and outbreaks in naïve areas. Pathog Glob Health 2014; 108(8): 349-55.
[http://dx.doi.org/10.1179/2047773214Y.0000000163] [PMID: 25491436]

[72]   Mercado-Reyes M, Acosta-Reyes J, Navarro-Lechuga E, *et al.* Dengue, chikungunya and zika virus coinfection: results of the national surveillance during the zika epidemic in Colombia. Epidemiol Infect 2019; 147: e77.
[http://dx.doi.org/10.1017/S095026881800359X] [PMID: 30869010]

[73]   Lin DCD, Weng SC, Tsao PN, Chu JJH, Shiao SH. Co-infection of dengue and Zika viruses mutually enhances viral replication in the mosquito *Aedes aegypti*. Parasit Vectors 2023; 16(1): 160.
[http://dx.doi.org/10.1186/s13071-023-05778-1] [PMID: 37165438]

[74]   Alsedig K, Eldigail MH, Elduma AH, *et al.* Prevalence of malaria and dengue co-infections among febrile patients during dengue transmission season in Kassala, eastern Sudan. PLoS Negl Trop Dis 2023; 17(10): e0011660.
[http://dx.doi.org/10.1371/journal.pntd.0011660] [PMID: 37792705]

[75]   Wiwanitkit V. Concurrent malaria and dengue infection: a brief summary and comment. Asian Pac J Trop Biomed 2011; 1(4): 326-7.
[http://dx.doi.org/10.1016/S2221-1691(11)60053-1] [PMID: 23569785]

[76]   Siddig EE, Mohamed NS, Ahmed A. Severe coinfection of dengue and malaria: A case report. Clin Case Rep 2024; 12(6): e9079.
[http://dx.doi.org/10.1002/ccr3.9079] [PMID: 38868112]

[77]   Vector-borne   diseases.   2024.   Available   from: https://www.who.int/news-room/fac-
-sheets/detail/vector-borne-diseases

[78]   Nuraini N, Fauzi IS, Fakhruddin M, Sopaheluwakan A, Soewono E. Climate-based dengue model in Semarang, Indonesia: Predictions and descriptive analysis. Infect Dis Model 2021; 6: 598-611.
[http://dx.doi.org/10.1016/j.idm.2021.03.005] [PMID: 33869907]

[79]   Varamballi P, Babu N N, Mudgal PP, *et al.* Spatial heterogeneity in the potential distribution of *Aedes* mosquitoes in India under current and future climatic scenarios. Acta Trop 2024; 260: 107403.
[http://dx.doi.org/10.1016/j.actatropica.2024.107403] [PMID: 39278522]

[80]   Abdullah NAMH, Dom NC, Salleh SA, Salim H, Precha N. The association between dengue case and climate: A systematic review and meta-analysis. One Health 2022; 15: 100452.
[http://dx.doi.org/10.1016/j.onehlt.2022.100452] [PMID: 36561711]

[81]   Bonnin L, Tran A, Herbreteau V, *et al.* Predicting the effects of climate change on dengue vector densities in southeast asia through process-based modeling. Environ Health Perspect 2022; 130(12): 127002.
[http://dx.doi.org/10.1289/EHP11068] [PMID: 36473499]

[82]   Nuraini N, Fauzi IS, Fakhruddin M, Sopaheluwakan A, Soewono E. Climate-based dengue model in Semarang, Indonesia: Predictions and descriptive analysis. Infect Dis Model 2021; 6: 598-611.
[http://dx.doi.org/10.1016/j.idm.2021.03.005] [PMID: 33869907]

[83]   Aguiar M, Anam V, Blyuss KB, *et al.* Mathematical models for dengue fever epidemiology: A 10-year systematic review. Phys Life Rev 2022; 40: 65-92.
[http://dx.doi.org/10.1016/j.plrev.2022.02.001] [PMID: 35219611]

[84]   Din A, Khan T, Li Y, Tahir H, Khan A, Khan WA. Mathematical analysis of dengue stochastic epidemic model. Results Phys 2021; 20: 103719.
[http://dx.doi.org/10.1016/j.rinp.2020.103719]

[85]   Jacintho L, Batista A, Ruas T, Marietto M, Silva F. An agent-based model for the spread of the dengue fever: A Swarm platform simulation approach. 2010; p. 2.
[http://dx.doi.org/10.1145/1878537.1878540]

[86]   Mahmood I, Jahan M, Groen D, Javed A, Shafait F. An agent-based simulation of the spread of dengue fever. Comput Sci ICCS 2020; 12139: 103-17.

[87]   Andraud M, Hens N, Marais C, Beutels P. Dynamic epidemiological models for dengue transmission: a systematic review of structural approaches. PLoS One 2012; 7(11): e49085.
[http://dx.doi.org/10.1371/journal.pone.0049085] [PMID: 23139836]

[88]   Pakaya R, Daniel D, Widayani P, Utarini A. Spatial model of Dengue Hemorrhagic Fever (DHF) risk: scoping review. BMC Public Health 2023; 23(1): 2448.
[http://dx.doi.org/10.1186/s12889-023-17185-3] [PMID: 38062404]

[89]   Side S, Rangkuti YM, Pane DG, Sinaga MS. Stability analysis susceptible, exposed, infected, recovered (SEIR) model for spread model for spread of dengue fever in medan. J Phys Conf Ser 2018; 954(1): 012018.
[http://dx.doi.org/10.1088/1742-6596/954/1/012018]

[90]   Catano-Lopez A, Rojas-Diaz D, Laniado H, Arboleda-Sánchez S, Puerta-Yepes ME, Lizarralde-Bejarano DP. An alternative model to explain the vectorial capacity using as example *Aedes aegypti* case in dengue transmission. Heliyon 2019; 5(10): e02577.
[http://dx.doi.org/10.1016/j.heliyon.2019.e02577] [PMID: 31687486]

[91]   Liu-Helmersson J, Stenlund H, Wilder-Smith A, Rocklöv J. Vectorial capacity of *Aedes aegypti*: effects of temperature and implications for global dengue epidemic potential. PLoS One 2014; 9(3): e89783.
[http://dx.doi.org/10.1371/journal.pone.0089783] [PMID: 24603439]

[92]   World Health Organization. Vector management and delivery of vector control services. Dengue: guidelines for diagnosis, treatment, prevention and control: new edition 2009. Available from: https://www.ncbi.nlm.nih.gov/books/NBK143163/

[93]   Pan American Health Organization. Vectors: Integrated management and public health entomology - PAHO/WHO | Pan American Health Organization. 2024. Available from: https://www.paho.org/en/topics/vectors-integrated-management-and-public-health-entomology

[94]   Mueller A, Thomas A, Brown J, *et al.* Geographic information system protocol for mapping areas targeted for mosquito control in North Carolina. PLoS One 2023; 18(3): e0278253.
[http://dx.doi.org/10.1371/journal.pone.0278253] [PMID: 36961789]

[95]   Caribbean Public Health Agency. CARPHA > VBD - Evaluation of New Vector Control Technologies. 2022 Available from: https://carpha.org/What-We-Do/VBD/Evaluation-of-New-V-ctor-Control-Technologies

CHAPTER 5

Climate Change and Malaria

Joel Jaison[1] and **Jayalakshmi Krishnan**[1,*]

[1] *Vector Biology Research Laboratory, Department of Biotechnology, Central University of Tamil Nadu, Thiruvarur, India*

Abstract: This chapter discusses the complex relationship between climate change and malaria, highlighting the deep impact of environmental shifts on vector-borne diseases. It begins by exploring the broader context of climate change and its influence on the distribution and intensity of vector-borne diseases globally. A key focus is on the impact of changing climate patterns on *Anopheles* mosquitoes, the primary vectors of malaria. The chapter examines how temperature, precipitation, and humidity variations affect mosquito behaviour, life cycle, and habitat suitability, consequently altering malaria transmission dynamics. The economic implications of these changes are analysed, emphasising the burden on healthcare systems and economies, particularly in vulnerable regions. The chapter also discusses the role of climate control and mitigation strategies in managing the spread of malaria. It outlines various interventions to reduce greenhouse gas emissions and improve adaptive capacities to mitigate the adverse effects of climate change on malaria prevalence. Disease surveillance is seen as a crucial component in this context, with an emphasis on the need for monitoring systems to track changes in disease patterns and vector populations. Innovative approaches and technologies for surveillance and data collection are presented, highlighting their importance in early detection and response to malaria outbreaks. This chapter provides current research and case studies and an overview of the challenges and opportunities in addressing the drastic effects of climate change and malaria. It emphasises the importance of integrated vector management strategies combining climate action with public health initiatives to reduce the spread of malaria.

Keywords: *Anopheles* mosquitoes, Case studies, Climate change, Climate control, Disease surveillance, Economic consequences, Malaria, Mitigation, Vector-borne diseases.

INTRODUCTION

Climate change, characterised by rising temperatures, altered precipitation patterns, and increasing frequency of harsh weather disasters, drastically affects

---

[*] **Corresponding author Jayalakshmi Krishnan:** Vector Biology Research Laboratory, Department of Biotechnology, Central University of Tamil Nadu, Thiruvarur, India; E-mail: jayalakshmi@cutn.ac.in

Jayalakshmi Krishnan, Sigamani Panneer, P. Thiyagarajan, Balachandar Vellingiri & Pradeep Kumar Srivastava (Eds.)

public health exponentially. One of the most concerning impacts is on the epidemiology of vector-borne diseases, notably malaria. Malaria, caused by the infestation of *Plasmodium* parasites and transmitted by *Anopheles* mosquitoes, remains a significant global health challenge [1]. As climate change alters the habitats and behaviours of these vectors, the dynamics of malaria transmission are shifting, necessitating innovative approaches in disease surveillance.

The phenomenon of climate change has now become a matter of global concern, compelling societies to confront the perils of global warming that place a burden on the planet. As the average global temperatures rise, driven by anthropogenic activities, such as the burning of fossil fuels, deforestation, and industrial processes, the resulting climatic shifts are becoming increasingly evident and severe [2]. The manifestations of these changes are varied and widespread: polar ice caps are melting at unprecedented rates, sea levels are rising, and extreme weather events, like hurricanes, droughts, and such, are becoming more frequent and intense. Here, we discuss the dynamics of these changes by examining the scientific principles influencing these shifts, the evidence supporting the urgent reality of global warming, and the impacts of these changes on ecosystems, economies, and human health. Furthermore, it explores the concept of disease spread, an area that encompasses both mitigation strategies aimed at finding the factors that accelerate the transmission of malaria and adaptation measures designed to combat these conditions that have already been observed in various regions. From international policies, such as the Paris Agreement, to technological innovations in disease surveillance, the chapter provides a comprehensive overview of the efforts being made to create a more sustainable, disease-free future. Understanding the correlation between natural events and human interventions becomes crucial as the world grapples with the challenges posed by climate change and public health. This exploration seeks not only to elucidate the current state of the climate crisis but also to inspire precautionary actions and collaborative solutions that can divert these devastating effects. This chapter aims to enlighten the readers with the knowledge necessary to engage in meaningful discourse and effective action in the fight against climate change through a detailed analysis of scientific data, policy frameworks, and emerging technologies.

Climate Change and Vector-borne Diseases

Climate change affects the spread of diseases, particularly vector-borne diseases, as the climatic conditions become more favourable for vectors, leading to an increased risk of disease transmission [3]. Vector-borne diseases are illnesses transmitted by vectors, such as mosquitoes, ticks, and fleas, which thrive in specific environmental conditions. One of the most significant impacts of climate change on vector-borne diseases is the expansion of the geographic range of vectors [4]. Warmer temperatures allow vectors to survive in areas where they previously could not, thereby exposing new populations to the diseases they carry [5]. For example, malaria, a disease transmitted by mosquitoes, is spreading at a higher rate due to global warming, putting millions of people at risk who were previously not affected.

Furthermore, climate change can alter the dynamics of vector populations, leading to increased breeding rates and shorter incubation periods for pathogens within the vectors, leading to concurrent and severe malaria outbreaks [6]. For instance, the Zika virus, primarily transmitted by *Aedes* mosquitoes, dramatically increased in recent years, partly due to changing climate patterns favouring mosquito breeding [7]. The impact of these changes on human health is profound, as isolated communities and tribals that were once protected from vector-borne diseases due to their remote locations are now facing new threats. Vulnerable populations, such as those living in poverty or with limited access to healthcare, are particularly at risk. However, the economic burden of treating these diseases and implementing vector control measures can also be significant, straining already overstretched healthcare systems.

Combatting the spread of vector-borne diseases during this period of intense climate change requires a holistic approach, as this is a multifactorial problem. Firstly, there needs to be a focus on mitigating climate change itself by reducing greenhouse gas emissions and transitioning to renewable energy sources. This will help slow down the drastic climate change and limit the extent of its impacts on vector populations. Secondly, efforts must be made to strengthen public health systems and improve access to healthcare, especially in vulnerable communities. This includes investing in disease surveillance, early detection, and response mechanisms to prevent outbreaks before they escalate.

Additionally, education and community engagement are crucial for raising awareness about the risks of vector-borne diseases and promoting preventative measures, such as insecticide-treated bed nets and mosquito repellents. Furthermore, Integrated Vector Management (IVM) strategies, including habitat modification, insecticide use, and biological control methods, can help reduce vector populations and minimise disease transmission [8]. These strategies should be tailored to local contexts and consider the specific environmental conditions causing vector proliferation.

Understanding the Impact of Climate Change on Malarial Mosquito Vectors

Malaria, a lethal mosquito-borne disease caused by the *Plasmodium* parasite, remains a disease challenge that the world is still dealing with [1]. Understanding the relationship between climate change and malaria transmission is critical in devising effective strategies for control [6, 9, 10]. Here, we examine how changes in temperature, rainfall patterns, and extreme weather events impact the distribution and life cycle of mosquitoes that carry the malaria parasite.

Temperature plays a significant role in aiding the life cycle and behaviour of mosquitoes, particularly those of the *Anopheles* genus, responsible for transmitting malaria [11]. As temperatures increase over a period due to climate change, the geographical range of these mosquitoes expands, bringing malaria to previously unaffected regions. Higher temperatures accelerate *Plasmodium* development within mosquitoes, reducing the time required for the parasite to mature and become infectious. Additionally, warmer temperatures can shorten the duration of the mosquito's life cycle, leading to increased breeding rates and higher mosquito populations as adaptations. Consequently, elevated temperatures create optimal environments for malaria transmission, heightening the risk of outbreaks in both endemic and non-endemic areas [12].

Alterations in rainfall patterns, another hallmark of climate change, impact mosquito breeding habitats and, consequently, malaria transmission dynamics [11]. While some regions may experience increased rainfall and flooding, others may face prolonged droughts. Both scenarios influence mosquito breeding habitats differently. Excessive rainfall can create stagnant water bodies ideal for mosquito larvae development, increasing mosquito populations. Conversely, droughts can form small, isolated water bodies, concentrating mosquito breeding sites and intensifying malaria transmission in affected areas. Moreover, changes in rainfall patterns can disrupt natural ecosystems, displacing mosquito predators and distributing the eggs through water, thereby altering the balance of vector populations.

Disastrous events, such as hurricanes, tornadoes, cyclones, and floods, are becoming more unpredictable and severe as the years pass due to climate change in recent years. These events not only cause immediate devastation but also have long-term implications for malaria transmission [13]. Floods, for instance, can displace communities, disrupt healthcare systems, and create breeding grounds for mosquitoes, leading to malaria outbreaks in affected areas [13]. Similarly, hurricanes and cyclones can weaken infrastructure and deter access to healthcare services, but the aftermath of such events often leads to socioeconomic losses, rendering affected regions more susceptible to malarial infections [14].

As temperatures continue to rise, weather patterns become increasingly unpredictable. Understanding the complex dynamics of mosquito vectors and malaria transmission is essential for effective prevention and control strategies.

Mitigating climate change through coordinated global efforts is crucial for preserving ecological balance and safeguarding public health against vector-borne diseases like malaria. By addressing the root causes of this climatic crisis and implementing adaptive measures, we can reduce the spread of malaria and protect susceptible populations from its devastating impact.

Malaria: A Global Concern

Protozoan parasites that come under the genus *Plasmodium* cause malaria and are a major cause of death and illness globally [1]. These parasites have been known to have a complex life cycle involving mosquito vectors and vertebrate hosts. The primary factors contributing to the re-emergence of malaria include the increase in drug-resistant strains of the parasite, the spread of insecticide-resistant mosquito strains, and the lack of effective licensed malaria vaccines [15, 16]. This chapter provides a summary of the disease, details about the parasite's life cycle, and information on the genome and proteome of *Plasmodium falciparum*, the species most lethal to humans, along with other recent developments in the field [17].

Malaria remains one of the most concerning public health topics globally, primarily influenced by the habitats and behaviours of its primary vectors: *Anopheles* mosquitoes [18]. These mosquitoes thrive in environments that provide ideal breeding and feeding conditions. As global climate patterns shift, driven by changing temperatures and precipitation patterns, the habitats of these vectors and consequently, the epidemiology of malaria, are undergoing profound transformations. Malaria is widespread in both the subtropics and tropics, with many tropical areas being endemic to the disease. Sub-Saharan Africa accounts for the majority of malaria cases, while other significant clusters are found in India, Brazil, Afghanistan, Sri Lanka, Thailand, Indonesia, Vietnam, Cambodia, and China [19, 20] (Fig. 1).

The term "malaria" comes from the Italian words '*mal-aria,*' meaning 'bad-air,' reflecting the early belief that the disease was associated with marshy areas [21]. In the late 19th century, French army surgeon Charles Louis Alphonse Laveran identified parasites in the blood of a malaria patient, and British medical officer Dr Ronald Ross in Hyderabad, India, discovered that mosquitoes transmit malaria [22]. Italian professor Giovanni Battista Grassi later determined that *Anopheles* mosquitoes exclusively transmit human malaria [23].

Malaria affects numerous countries, with reports indicating between 350 and 500 million cases in 2004 [24]. Over two billion people, or more than 40% of the worldwide population, are at risk of contracting malaria [25]. According to World Health Organization (WHO) reports, from 1999 to 2004, the annual death toll from malaria was estimated at 1.1 to 1.3 million [26]. Malaria costs Africa over

$12 billion annually and is responsible for about 25% of all deaths in children under the age of five on the continent [27]. Public health measures and economic development have nearly or completely eliminated the disease in many temperate regions, such as Western Europe and the USA, except for cases that migrated through international travel.

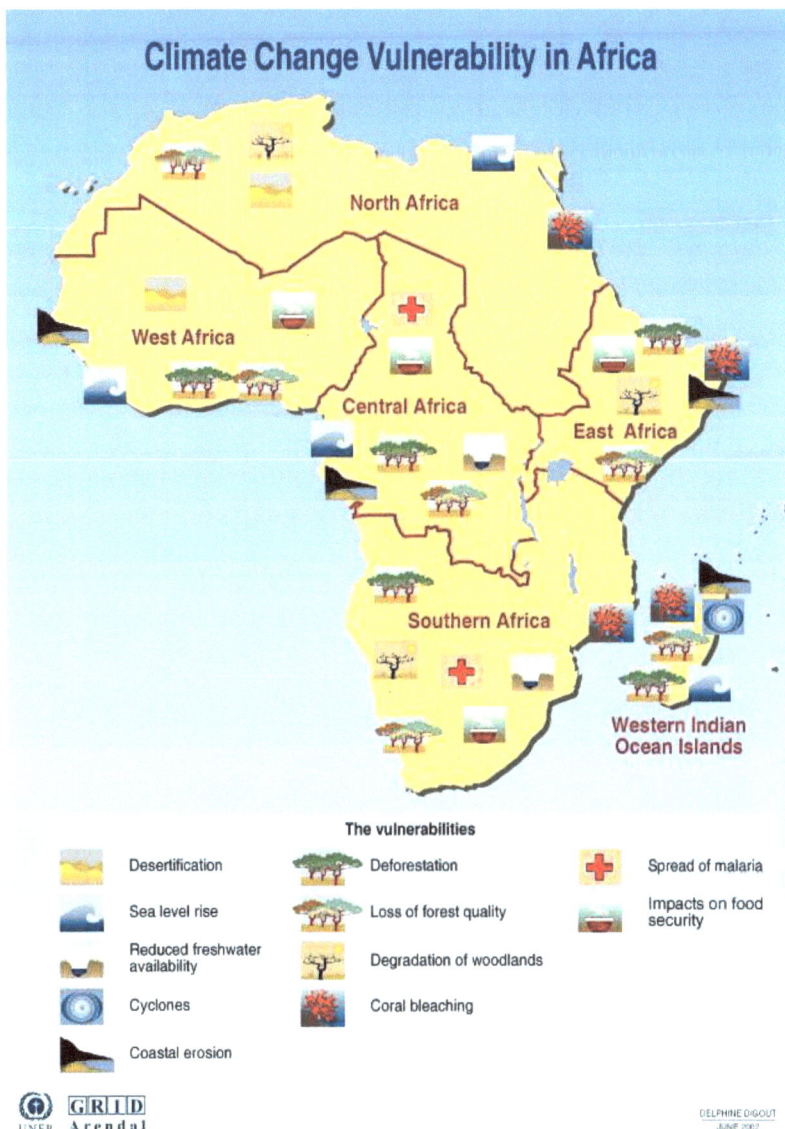

Fig. (1). Climate change vulnerability map of the African subcontinent, showing areas where malaria spread is potential (indicated by red crosses). Source: Delphine *Digout, Revised by Hugo Ahlenius, UNEP/GRID-Arendal*https://www.grida.no/resources/6895.

Malaria is a concerning health risk, with an estimated 229 million reported cases globally in 2019, predominantly in the African region, where 94% of these cases occurred [28]. Despite efforts to control and eradicate malaria over the past century, progress has been slow, with a recent rise in malaria incidence observed in various regions since 2014, indicating stunted progress [17]. This increase in cases shows the urgent need for new antimalarial drugs with novel, unique mechanisms of action, as resistance to current front-line therapies and drugs has emerged. The management of malaria involves both preventive approaches, with early diagnosis and effective treatment being crucial to prevent the progression of mild malaria to more dangerous, severe forms of the disease. To neutralise the spread of antimalarial drug resistance, the World Health Organization (WHO) recommends the use of combination therapy with at least two effective antimalarial agents that have different mechanisms of action for all episodes of malaria.

Anopheles stephensi: A Unique and Expanding Urban Malaria Vector

Anopheles stephensi is a significant vector of human malaria, responsible for transmitting malaria parasites in numerous countries across Southeast Asia, the Middle East, and the Arabian Peninsula [29]. Unlike most malaria vectors that thrive in rural settings, *Anopheles stephensi* has adapted to survive in urban and semi-urban environments, marking it as a unique and formidable challenge in the fight against malaria [30] (Fig. **2**). This adaptability has led to its recent spread to different parts of Africa, raising concerns about potential outbreaks of urban malaria and complicating existing control and elimination efforts in Africa [30].

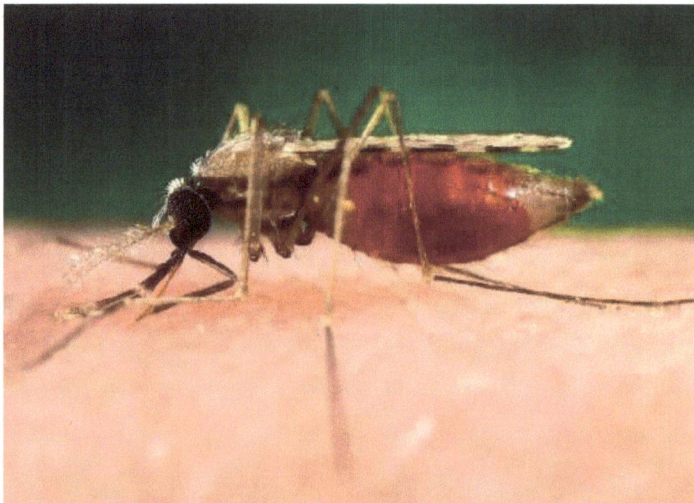

Fig. (2). *Blood-fed Malaria vector -Anopheles minimus* (Source: James Gathany, Center for Disease Control and Prevention).

Historically, *Anopheles stephensi* has been prevalent in urban regions of Southeast Asia, the Middle East, and the Arabian Peninsula [29]. However, its geographical range has recently extended into East Africa [30]. First reported in Djibouti in 2012, the mosquito was subsequently found in Ethiopia in 2016, Sudan in 2018, and Somalia in 2019 [9, 30 - 32]. This expansion is alarming as it poses a new threat to malaria control in urban African settings where 40% of sub-Saharan Africans live.

Anopheles stephensi exhibits three distinct biological forms: type, intermediate, and mysorensis, distinguishable by egg morphology [33]. The type and intermediate forms are efficient malaria vectors, whereas the mysorensis form is primarily zoophilic, preferring animal blood and thus playing a lesser role in malaria transmission [34]. In urban environments, the type form is anthropophilic, endophagic, and endophilic, often breeding in artificial containers such as water barrels and cisterns. Conversely, in rural settings, themysorensis form is zoophilic and exophilic, with juveniles found in natural water bodies like irrigation canals and stream pools [35].

Anopheles stephensi is small to medium-sized, light brown to grey, and divided into three main regions: head, thorax, and abdomen. The head parts comprise compound eyes, antennae, sensory palps, and a proboscis for feeding. The thoracic region, equipped with legs and wings, is the locomotive unit, featuring pale spots on the wings and pale bands on the palps [36]. The abdomen, involved in digestion and reproduction, can expand significantly during blood feeding. *Anopheles stephensi* is a highly competent vector for malaria parasites, notably *Plasmodium falciparum* and *Plasmodium vivax*. These parasites can cause severe illness and death, particularly in children under five [37]. The presence of *Anopheles stephensi* in urban African settings, previously considered mostly free of such vectors, may lead to a resurgence of malaria, as seen in Djibouti [30].

The spread of *Anopheles stephensi* to Africa complicates malaria control efforts due to its unique behavioural and ecological traits [30]. Effective malaria control requires understanding the mosquito's bionomics in Africa, including insecticide resistance, feeding and resting behaviours, susceptibility to parasite infection and transmission, and habitat preferences. The potential for this mosquito to thrive in urban environments, where traditional malaria control measures may be less effective, necessitates re-evaluating current strategies. Several management practices can mitigate the risk of malaria transmission by *Anopheles stephensi*. These include environmental modifications to eliminate breeding sites, community education to increase awareness and promote preventive behaviors, and the use of insecticide-treated bed nets and indoor residual spraying.

Additionally, spatial repellents and biological control methods can be employed [8].

Anopheles stephensi represents a unique challenge in the global fight against malaria, particularly due to its adaptability to urban environments and recent geographic expansion. Its presence in Africa could significantly impact malaria transmission dynamics, making it crucial to understand its behaviour, resistance patterns, and ecological preferences [30]. Effective malaria control and elimination will depend on tailored strategies addressing the specific threats this vector poses in diverse environments.

Life Cycle of *Anopheles* Mosquitoes

The life cycle of *Anopheles* mosquitoes, the primary vectors of malaria, is a complex process consisting of four distinct stages of development: egg, larva, pupa, and adult. Each stage is adapted to the mosquito's aquatic and terrestrial environments, ensuring their survival and propagation.

Eggs

The life cycle of *Anopheles* mosquitoes begins with the laying of eggs by adult females. These mosquitoes use marshy areas or the banks of shallow creeks and streams for egg-laying, as these environments provide the necessary moisture [38, 39]. Unlike other mosquito species, *Anopheles* females lay their eggs directly on the water surface. These eggs are laid one at a time and float due to specialized structures that prevent them from sinking [38]. Each female can lay between 50 and 200 eggs at a time, maximizing the potential for survival of the eggs due to their large number [18]. However, these eggs are highly sensitive to desiccation and cannot survive drying out [39]. Therefore, selecting an appropriate aquatic habitat is crucial for the development of the eggs and the subsequent stages of the mosquito's life cycle.

Larvae

The mosquito larvae, commonly known as 'wrigglers', emerge and begin their aquatic life upon hatching. *Anopheles* larvae are uniquely adapted to their aquatic setting. They possess specialised breathing organs called spiracles on their abdomen, allowing them to breathe atmospheric oxygen while remaining submerged [40]. This adaptation enables them to survive underwater while minimising exposure to predators. During the larval stage, these mosquitoes undergo four moults, shedding their exoskeletons as they grow [18]. Each moult signifies a new instar, a developmental phase that brings the larva closer to maturity. The larval feed consists of microorganisms and organic matter in the water, accumulating the energy required for the next stage of their life cycle.

Pupae

After completing the larval stages, *Anopheles* mosquitoes enter the pupal stage, which also occurs in water. The pupae, often called 'tumblers' due to their tumbling motion when disturbed, do not feed during this stage. Unlike the larvae, pupae do not possess external mouthparts and thus remain inactive in terms of feeding [41]. However, the pupal stage is a period of intense and rigorous transformation. Inside the pupal casing, the mosquito undergoes metamorphosis, reorganising its body structure to emerge as an adult. The pupae float below the water's surface, allowing the emerging adult mosquito to access the air and prepare for its final transformation.

Adults

The adult stage marks the final stage of the mosquito's life cycle. Upon emerging from the pupal casing, the adult mosquito is fully formed and capable of flight. Female *Anopheles* mosquitoes, in particular, play a crucial role in malaria transmission. They seek out blood meals from humans and animals, typically late at night, as blood is essential for the development of their eggs. After feeding, female mosquitoes rest for a few days to digest the blood and develop their eggs [36]. They often seek out dark, sheltered areas for resting during the daytime. Once the eggs are fully developed, the female returns to water sources to lay them, thus continuing the cycle. Male *Anopheles* mosquitoes primarily feed on nectar and other plant juices [42]. Males often gather in large swarms around dusk, engaging in mating flights [41]. Females join these swarms to mate, ensuring the propagation of their species. Interestingly, *Anopheles* mosquitoes have limited flight ranges, generally not flying more than 1.2 miles (2 kilometres) from their larval habitats [43]. This limited mobility implies the importance of suitable aquatic environments for their reproductive success.

The life cycle of *Anopheles* mosquitoes is a remarkable journey from egg to adult, each stage entangled with different adaptations to water and each adaptation finely tuned to ensure survival and reproduction. Understanding this life cycle is crucial in understanding how climate controls the survival of these species, as it highlights potential intervention points where control measures can be most effective. By disrupting the mosquito's life cycle at various stages, it is possible to reduce their populations and limit the spread of malaria.

Parasitic Development of *Plasmodium*

Malaria transmission begins when an infected female *Anopheles* mosquito bites the human host [44]. Out of the approximately 400 species of *Anopheles* worldwide, around 60 serve as malaria vectors under natural conditions, with 30 of significant importance. Malaria parasites are eukaryotic single-celled microorganisms belonging to the genus *Plasmodium* [45]. While more than 100 species of *Plasmodium* can infect various animals, including reptiles, birds, and mammals, only four species naturally infect humans: *Plasmodium falciparum*, *Plasmodium vivax*, *Plasmodium ovale*, and *Plasmodium malariae* [17, 45]. These four species differ in morphology, immunology, geographical distribution, relapse patterns, and drug responses. *P. falciparum* is the deadliest, causing severe malaria and is the leading cause of malaria deaths in young children in Africa [32]. *P. ovale*, the least common, is mainly found in West Africa, while *P. malariae* has a worldwide but low-frequency presence. *P. vivax* is the most widespread but rarely fatal. Both *P. falciparum* and *P. vivax* can cause severe anaemia, but it is more deadly in *P. falciparum* infections, particularly among African children, due to severe blood loss and potential cerebral malaria, a fatal condition where infected erythrocytes obstruct brain blood vessels [46]. Additionally, *P. ovale* and *P. vivax* have dormant liver stages called hypnozoites, which can remain inactive for weeks to years, leading to malaria relapses [47]. *P. malariae* can cause long-lasting blood-stage infections that, if untreated, may persist asymptomatically for several decades.

Malarial parasites have a complex life cycle that requires specialised protein expression for survival in both the invertebrate and vertebrate hosts. These proteins are essential for both intracellular and extracellular survival, enabling the parasites to invade various cell types and evade host immune responses. Upon entering the human host, *P. falciparum* and *P. malariae* sporozoites trigger immediate schizogony, while *P. ovale* and *P. vivax* sporozoites can either trigger immediate schizogony or undergo delayed schizogony *via* the hypnozoite stage [21]. The life cycle of the malaria parasite includes several stages, beginning with the entry of sporozoites into the bloodstream.

Infective sporozoites from the *Anopheles* mosquito's salivary gland are injected into the human host, along with saliva that contains anticoagulants, facilitating a smooth blood meal [48]. While it was previously believed that sporozoites quickly disperse from the injection site, a recent study using the rodent parasite *Plasmodium yoelii* indicates that most sporozoites remain at the injection site for hours, gradually entering the bloodstream [49]. Once in the human bloodstream, *Plasmodium falciparum* sporozoites reach the liver, where they invade hepatocytes and remain for 9-16 days, undergoing asexual replication in a process known as exo-erythrocytic schizogony. The precise mechanisms for targeting and invading hepatocytes are not fully understood; however, it is known that sporozoite migration through multiple hepatocytes is crucial for completing the life cycle [50]. The sporozoites use receptors, primarily thrombospondin domains on the circumsporozoite protein and thrombospondin-related adhesive protein, to bind specifically to heparan sulfate proteoglycans on hepatocytes. Each sporozoite can produce tens of thousands of merozoites within a hepatocyte, and each merozoite can subsequently invade a red blood cell upon release from the liver. Studies with rodent malaria parasites, such as *Plasmodium berghei*, have shown that liver-stage parasites manipulate host cells to ensure the safe delivery of merozoites into the bloodstream, with hepatocyte-derived merosomes acting as protective shuttles [50, 51]. The duration of the tissue phase, known as the prepatent period, varies by species, ranging from 8-25 days for *P. falciparum*, 8-27 days for *P. vivax*, 9-17 days for *P. ovale*, and 15-30 days for *P. malariae* [52].

Merozoites invade erythrocytes through a complex process consisting of four phases: initial recognition and reversible attachment to the erythrocyte membrane; reorientation and junction formation at the merozoite's apical end, accompanied by the release of substances from rhoptries and micronemes to form the parasitophorous vacuole; movement of the junction and invagination of the erythrocyte membrane, with the removal of the merozoite's surface coat; and the resealing of the vacuole and erythrocyte membranes upon invasion completion [49]. Due to the specific molecular interactions required for this process, it is an attractive target for malaria intervention strategies. Inside the erythrocyte, asexual division begins, with the parasite progressing through different stages. The early trophozoite, often called the 'ring form' due to its morphology, enlarges and exhibits active metabolism, including glucose glycolysis, ingestion of host cytoplasm, and haemoglobin proteolysis into amino acids [53]. The toxic heme by-product is polymerised into hemozoin and stored within the food vacuoles. Multiple rounds of nuclear division without cytokinesis mark the end of the trophic stage, forming schizonts, which release about 20 merozoites upon erythrocyte lysis, continuing the cycle every 48 hours for *P. falciparum*, *P. ovale*, and *P. vivax*, and every 72 hours for *P. malariae*. This synchronous release triggers immune responses, causing characteristic clinical symptoms. Specific ligand-receptor interactions have been identified as essential for invasion, with genetic disruptions leading to shifts in alternative pathways. The *P. falciparum* genome reveals that invasion molecules are part of larger gene families, with Merozoite Surface Proteins (MSPs) playing a crucial role [54]. EBA-175, a protein similar to *P. vivax*'s Duffy antigen-binding proteins, binds to glycophorin A on erythrocytes [55]. Post-invasion, PfEMP1, encoded by the var gene family, is expressed on infected erythrocytes and is key to pathogenesis and immune evasion, with only one var gene expressed at a time within infected cells [56].

Recent studies have identified epigenetic marks associated with silenced var genes, providing advantages in pathogenesis and immune evasion [57, 58]. A small number of merozoites differentiate into gametocytes, essential for transmission through *Anopheles* mosquitoes. In *P. falciparum*, gametocytogenesis takes 10-12 days, with gametocytes appearing 5 to 23 days post-primary attack in *P. malariae* infections [59].

When a mosquito feeds on an infected individual, it may ingest gametocytes into its midgut. Here, macrogametocytes develop into macrogametes, and ex-flagellation of microgametocytes produces microgametes. These gametes fuse and undergo fertilisation to form a zygote, which then transforms into an ookinete. The ookinete penetrates the midgut cell wall and develops into an oocyst [49]. Recent research has shown that the gamete surface antigen Pfs230 mediates the binding of human red blood cells to ex-flagellating male parasites, forming clusters known as ex-flagellation centers, from which individual motile microgametes are released [60]. This protein is crucial for oocyst development, a vital step in the transmission of malaria. Sporogony within the oocyst generates numerous sporozoites, which migrate to the salivary glands once the oocyst ruptures. These sporozoites reach the salivary glands after 10-18 days, rendering the mosquito infective for 1-2 months [48]. The *Plasmodium* life cycle recommences when this infected mosquito bites a susceptible host [44].

Diagnosis, Treatment, and Prevention

The accumulation and sequestration of parasite-infected Red Blood Cells (RBCs) in organs such as the heart, brain, lungs, kidneys, subcutaneous tissues, and placenta are hallmarks of *P. falciparum* infection [37]. This sequestration results from interactions between parasite-derived proteins on the surfaces of infected RBCs and host molecules on uninfected RBCs, endothelial cells, and, in some cases, placental cells [61]. Specific receptors like hyaluronic acid and Chondroitin Sulfate A (CSA) in placental infections and Intercellular Adhesion Molecule 1 (ICAM-1) in cerebral malaria facilitate parasite adhesion [62 - 64]. Malaria symptoms can emerge as early as 6-8 days post-infection or months after leaving a malarial area, including fever, shivering, cough, respiratory distress, joint pain, headache, diarrhoea, vomiting, and convulsions. Severe malaria, often characterised by jaundice, kidney failure, and severe anaemia, can be fatal [64]. Although many malaria cases are non-life-threatening, the triggers for severe disease are not yet fully understood [65]. Malaria poses a significant risk to pregnant women and young children, contributing to perinatal mortality in endemic regions. Placental sequestration of *P. falciparum* can lead to adverse outcomes like premature delivery, low birth weight, and increased neonatal mortality. Immunity to pregnancy-associated malaria gradually develops with repeated exposure, making multi-gravid women less susceptible than primigravid women [59]. Diagnosis combines clinical observations, patient history, and diagnostic tests, primarily microscopic blood examination [66]. Rapid diagnostic tests detect malaria antigens quickly but are relatively costly and cannot distinguish between *P. ovale, P. malariae,* and *P. vivax* [67]. Although three consecutive negative tests can typically rule out malaria, prompt and adequate treatment can still cure the disease. Historically, quinine was the first widely used treatment, but resistance to common drugs like Fansidar and chloroquine has emerged [68]. Combination therapy, using drugs such as artemisinin and its derivatives like artesunate or artemether, is now standard to combat resistance. Despite the absence of a clinically approved malaria vaccine, several are in development. Global initiatives, such as the WHO's Roll Back Malaria program and the Global Fund to Fight AIDS, Tuberculosis, and Malaria, aim to reduce malaria transmission through drug treatment, vaccination, and vector control [69]. A novel approach involves genetically modifying mosquitoes to be refractory to malaria transmission. Advances in germ-line transformation, tissue-specific promoters, and effector molecules have produced transgenic mosquitoes that do not transmit malaria. However, these genetically modified mosquitoes must thrive and compete with wild types in the field for long-term success. Recent studies suggest that transgenic mosquitoes may have a fitness advantage over wild types when fed blood infected with *Plasmodium,* but further research is needed to ensure their stability and effectiveness in natural settings [70].

Effect of Temperature on *Anopheles* Mosquito Population Dynamics

We will discuss a study on how changes in temperature affect the mosquito population in this section [12]. The researchers of this study employed a sophisticated approach by developing a temperature-dependent, stage-structured delayed differential equation model. This model was specifically designed to elucidate how climatic variations influence mosquito population dynamics and, consequently, the transmission of malaria. By structuring the model around the different developmental stages of mosquitoes, the study aimed to capture the often-forgotten effects of temperature on mosquito life cycles and their capacity to spread malaria [12].

Local Sensitivity Analysis

To identify the factors that most significantly impact mosquito populations and their ability to transmit malaria, a local sensitivity analysis was conducted. This analysis examined twelve different parameters within the model across a temperature range from 16 to 40°C. The purpose was to determine how sensitive these parameters were to changes in temperature and how this sensitivity affected key outcomes, such as larval and adult mosquito abundance, recruitment into the adult stage, and the number of mosquitoes capable of transmitting malaria [12].

Model Parameter Estimation

The model incorporated several critical parameters that govern the development rate of mosquitoes through their various life stages: egg, larva, pupa, and adult. These parameters, labelled as a and b, were empirically derived and represented the influence of temperature on these developmental rates. The model could more accurately simulate real-world mosquito population dynamics under varying temperature conditions by accurately estimating these parameters [12].

Data Analysis

Comprehensive data analysis was conducted to assess the impact of temperature on mosquito populations and their potential to transmit malaria. This analysis involved comparing model predictions with experimental data to understand how temperature variations affected the population dynamics and the transmission potential of malaria-carrying mosquitoes [12].

Model Validation

The accuracy and reliability of the model were likely ensured through rigorous validation against empirical data. This step was crucial for confirming that the model could reliably predict malaria risk under different temperature scenarios, thereby enhancing its practical utility in forecasting and mitigating malaria outbreaks [9].

The research revealed that mosquito population dynamics, especially the number of mosquitoes capable of transmitting malaria, are highly sensitive to temperature changes. This sensitivity is primarily due to the temperature-dependent rates of development during the juvenile stages of mosquitoes. The study emphasized that detailed vector biology must be incorporated into predictive models to accurately reflect the impacts of temperature on mosquito populations and malaria transmission. By integrating the entire mosquito life cycle into the temperature-dependent model, the researchers achieved more precise predictions of peak mosquito abundance related to malaria transmission. This understanding highlights the importance of considering temperature effects when forecasting malaria risk, leading to more informed strategies for malaria control and prevention.

The practical implications of this study included the following:

- ***Enhanced Malaria Control Strategies***: Understanding the temperature sensitivity of *Anopheles* mosquito population dynamics and malaria transmission can help to develop more specific and effective control strategies. By considering temperature fluctuations, interventions can be timed and tailored to reduce mosquito populations and malaria transmission rates. This approach enables a more precise implementation of control measures, potentially enhancing their efficacy.
- ***Improved Malaria Risk Prediction***: The findings emphasise the importance of incorporating detailed vector biology, including temperature effects, into predictive models for malaria risk assessment. This can lead to more precise predictions of peak mosquito abundance and, consequently, better forecasting of malaria outbreaks. Accurate predictions are crucial for timely and effective public health responses to potential malaria surges.
- ***Climate Change Adaptation***: With climate change influencing temperature patterns, this research signifies the need to adapt malaria control measures to changing environmental conditions. By understanding how temperature impacts mosquito populations and malaria transmission, public health interventions can be adjusted to mitigate the effects of climate change on the malaria burden. This proactive approach is necessary for enhancing the effectiveness of malaria control in a world where rising temperatures have become a matter of concern.
- ***Targeted Mosquito Control***: The temperature-dependent model developed in the study can inform targeted mosquito control efforts. By identifying temperature-sensitive stages in the mosquito life cycle, interventions can focus on disrupting these critical developmental phases to reduce mosquito abundance and limit malaria transmission. This targeted strategy enhances the efficiency and effectiveness of mosquito control programs, potentially reducing the overall malaria burden.

Climate Change Impacts Malaria in Africa: An Analysis of Vector Redistribution

Malaria remains one of the direst health challenges in Africa, significantly affecting both mortality and morbidity rates across the continent [30]. This disease, caused by the *Plasmodium* parasite and transmitted by *Anopheles* mosquitoes, greatly affects public health systems and hinders socio-economic development. As climate change continues to change present environmental conditions, there is a rising concern about its potential impact on the distribution of vector-borne diseases like malaria. This section explores a study on how climate change might influence the geographical redistribution of *Anopheles* mosquitoes, specifically *Anopheles gambiae* and *Anopheles arabiensis*, and discusses the implications for malaria control strategies throughout Africa [6]. Climate change is expected to have a considerable impact on the epidemiology of vector-borne diseases. Changes in temperature, rainfall patterns, and humidity can affect the lifecycle and habitat suitability of disease vectors, leading to shifts in their geographical distribution [12, 71]. For malaria, the *Anopheles* mosquito vectors are highly sensitive to these climatic factors. Increased temperatures can accelerate the mosquito lifecycle and enhance parasite development, while altered rainfall patterns can create new breeding sites or render existing ones unsuitable.

The primary aim of this study is to predict and map the potential redistribution of *Anopheles* mosquitoes in Africa using existing entomological data. By developing models based on CLIMEX parameters, the study estimates the geographical distribution and seasonal abundance of these mosquitoes under various climate change scenarios. CLIMEX is a simulation tool used to predict the dynamic distribution of species based on certain climatic factors. In this study, parameters such as temperature, rainfall, and humidity were calibrated to understand how future climate conditions might influence the distribution of *Anopheles gambiae* and *Anopheles arabiensis* [6, 71].

Anopheles gambiae and *Anopheles arabiensis* are the primary vectors of malaria in Africa. Understanding their potential shifts in geographical boundaries is crucial for effective malaria control. These species have different ecological preferences and behaviours, making it essential to study them separately under various climate change scenarios. The models predict that climate change could lead to significant shifts in the geographical range of these vectors, which in turn would affect malaria transmission patterns across the continent [6].

The study predicts notable changes in the geographical boundaries of *Anopheles* mosquitoes. In some regions, suitable habitats for these mosquitoes are expected to expand, while in others, they may contract or expand depending on various conditions. For instance, areas that become warmer and wetter might see an increase in mosquito populations, thereby elevating the risk of malaria transmission. On the contrary, regions that experience extreme temperatures or reduced rainfall may become less suitable for mosquito breeding, which could potentially reduce malaria prevalence. These shifts underscore the importance of awareness and preparation for potential changes in vector distribution, enabling effective planning and implementation of malaria control strategies [6].

The findings of this study have several practical implications for malaria control in Africa. By predicting and mapping the potential redistribution of *Anopheles* mosquitoes, the research provides valuable insights for policymakers, public health officials, and researchers. These insights are crucial for the development of early warning systems to anticipate changes in malaria vector distribution due to climate change. Early warning systems can enhance preparedness and allow for timely interventions, such as targeted vector control measures and resource allocation.

Development of Targeted Interventions

The models developed in this study can help in the formulation and implementation of targeted interventions to control malaria vectors effectively. By understanding the seasonal abundance and potential distribution of *Anopheles* mosquitoes under different climate change scenarios, health officials can prioritise areas for intervention and optimise the use of resources. This targeted approach is essential for managing limited resources and maximising the impact of control measures.

Strategic Planning and Resource Allocation

Understanding the possible future geographical range of malaria vectors and the disease itself enables strategic planning and resource distribution. Public health programs can be tailored to address the specific needs of regions likely to experience changes in vector distribution. This strategic planning is vital for ensuring that control measures are sustainable and effective in the long term. It also allows for the implementation of adaptive options to recognise the impacts of climate change on malaria transmission.

Enhancing Malaria Control Programs

The results of the study are valuable for enhancing malaria control programs at various levels. By providing evidence-based insights, the research supports decision-making processes and helps to improve the effectiveness of control efforts. For example, the findings can inform the development of policies and strategies that integrate climate change adaptation into malaria control programs. This integration is crucial for building resilient health systems capable of responding to the dynamic challenges posed by climate change.

The study emphasises the crucial role of climate crisis in the distribution of *Anopheles* mosquitoes in Africa and the subsequent implications for malaria transmission. By predicting and mapping the potential redistribution of these vectors, the research offers valuable insights for planning and implementing effective malaria control strategies. As mentioned earlier, understanding the potential shifts in geographical boundaries of *Anopheles gambiae* and *Anopheles arabiensis* is crucial for developing targeted interventions, enhancing preparedness, and ensuring sustainable malaria control in the face of climate change [6]. The findings emphasise the importance of proactive measures and evidence-based decision-making in addressing the challenges posed by changing disease dynamics. As climate change continues to evolve, ongoing research and adaptive strategies will be essential for safeguarding public health and reducing the burden of malaria in Africa.

Analysis of Economic Consequences

Malaria remains a significant and widespread health concern, particularly affecting populations in developing countries, where its impact extends beyond public health to the nation's economy. Here, we aim to understand the correlation between the spread of malaria and its repercussions on a country's economy, with a specific focus on changing patterns, climate change influences, healthcare costs, and productivity losses.

The dynamic nature of malaria transmission patterns significantly influences economic stability, particularly in developing countries. As malaria prevalence fluctuates due to factors, such as vector control measures, population movement, and socioeconomic changes, the national economy bears the weight and strain of these shifts [72]. In regions where malaria incidence is high, healthcare deals with diagnosis, treatment, and prevention efforts, thereby diverting resources away from other essential health services. Moreover, households affected by malaria often face increased healthcare expenditure, leading to financial strain and potential impoverishment. Furthermore, losing household income due to illness or caring for sick family members can lead to poverty and hinder economic development. In agricultural settings where malaria is endemic, productivity declines as workers fall ill, reducing agricultural yields and leading to economic losses for individuals and communities.

Climate change significantly impacts the distribution and intensity of malaria transmission, thereby complicating its economic implications. Shifts in temperature and precipitation patterns change the favourability of the habitat for malaria vectors, expanding the geographical range of transmission and intensifying outbreaks in previously unaffected areas [11]. This phenomenon increases healthcare costs and strains economies unprepared for the emergence of malaria. Furthermore, the economic implications of climate-induced malaria spread extend to sectors such as agriculture and tourism [73]. Tourism, hailed as a vital industry for many developing countries, suffers as travellers avoid destinations deemed high-risk for malaria transmission. Agricultural productivity faces additional challenges as changing climate patterns disrupt traditional farming practices, increasing the vulnerability of crops to pests and diseases and thereby increasing the likelihood of co-infections in malaria-affected patients.

Addressing the economic toll of malaria requires an approach that combines robust healthcare systems, targeted interventions, and adaptation strategies to combat the effects of climate change [73]. Investing in malaria control measures, such as vector control, early diagnosis, and effective treatment, saves lives and reduces the economic burden associated with the disease. Additionally, strengthening health systems to improve access to quality healthcare services ensures timely diagnosis and treatment, preventing illness-related productivity losses. Furthermore, building resilience to climate change is crucial in reducing the economic instability of populations due to a hike in malaria cases. Implementing climate-conscious agricultural practices, enhancing water resource management, and promoting sustainable land use can mitigate the environmental drivers of malaria while fostering economic sustainability [74]. Additionally, integrating malaria control efforts with broader development agendas, such as poverty reduction and infrastructure development, can enhance the stability of the economy and promote inclusive economic growth.

The spread of malaria poses a significant socioeconomic challenge, particularly for developing countries already grappling with resource constraints and climate-related events. By investing in robust healthcare systems, climate adaptation measures, and integrated development approaches, policymakers can mitigate the economic toll of malaria and pave the way for sustainable and resilient economies.

Vaccines for Malaria Prevention: A Recent Development

Malaria has been a global concern for a long time due to the lack of feasible vaccinations. However, the WHO recently approved and recommended a second vaccine, following the RTS, S/AS01 vaccine [75]. A beacon of hope emerged with the World Health Organization's (WHO) recommendation of a new vaccine, the R21/Matrix-M [76]. We will see the significance of this milestone, its implications, and the journey towards a malaria-free future in this section.

The announcement of the WHO's recommendation for the R21/Matrix-M vaccine marked a milestone in the fight against malaria [76]. Backed by the Strategic Advisory Group of Experts on Immunization (SAGE) and the Malaria Policy Advisory Group (MPAG), this decision was made after rigorous evaluation and analysis. Such a decision was made during the WHO's regular biannual meeting from September 25th to 29th. It shed light on the current scenario of a broader spectrum of diseases, including dengue and meningitis, alongside crucial insights into immunisation schedules and product recommendations for combating COVID-19.

The R21/Matrix-M vaccine became the second WHO-recommended malaria vaccine, following in the footsteps of the RTS, S/AS01 vaccine, which earned its recommendation in 2021. These vaccines have been proven safe and effective against malaria in both children and adults [77]. Given the toll malaria takes on African children, where nearly half a million lives are claimed by the disease annually, the arrival of these vaccines ushered in a new era of hope and resilience.

The demand for malaria vaccines increased, emphasising the need to close the gap between supply and demand. While the supply of RTS,S remained limited, including R21 in the WHO's arsenal of recommended vaccines promised to compensate for this scarcity. This would help African rural populations dealing with intense climatic changes in the African subcontinent gain immunity against malaria. With the potential to narrow the demand-and-supply gap, the deployment of these vaccines will offer a lifeline to countless children at risk of malaria's deadly embrace.

The R21/Matrix-M vaccine boasted several key attributes, making it a potent weapon against malaria. Evidence from clinical trials of the vaccine demonstrated high efficacy, particularly when administered just before the peak malaria transmission season [75, 77]. Its impact extended beyond seasonal contexts, demonstrating robust efficacy across various transmission settings. At least 28 African countries have signed to integrate the WHO-recommended malaria vaccine into their national immunisation programs to bring mass immunisation to the sub-continent. In the annals of global health, the WHO's recommendation of the R21/Matrix-M vaccine marked a milestone in vaccines against malaria.

Control and Prevention Strategies in the Context of Climate Change

Climate change is increasingly shaping the landscape of malaria control and prevention. Rising temperatures, changes in precipitation patterns, and ecological disturbances are modifying the distribution and behaviour of mosquitoes, thereby affecting the efficiency of existing control measures [11]. Here, we discuss climate change and malaria, examining its implications for current control strategies and proposing adaptive measures to combat the evolving threat.

Climate change exerts different effects on malaria transmission dynamics. Warmer temperatures accelerate malaria parasite development within mosquitoes, shortening the incubation period and potentially increasing transmission rates. Moreover, altered precipitation patterns can create breeding habitats crucial to mosquito proliferation, expanding the geographic range of malaria transmission [11]. Temperature and humidity changes also influence mosquitoes' survival and biting behaviour, leading to shifts in their spatial distribution and peak activity periods [71].

The evolving climate poses challenges to conventional malaria control strategies. Insecticide-treated bed nets and indoor residual spraying, which have been pivotal in reducing malaria incidence, may become less effective as mosquitoes adapt to changing environmental conditions [8]. Additionally, the emergence of insecticide resistance among mosquito populations further complicates vector control efforts. Climate-driven alterations in mosquito behaviour and habitat suitability necessitate a reassessment of the spatial and temporal targeting of control interventions.

Adaptive strategies must be devised and implemented to confront the evolving threat of malaria under climate change. Integrated Vector Management (IVM) approaches, which combine various control measures tailored to local epidemiological and environmental conditions, offer a flexible framework for adaptation [8]. This includes deploying novel vector control tools, such as larvicidal agents, spatial repellents, and genetic modification techniques, which can complement existing interventions and mitigate the impact of climate-induced changes.

Furthermore, enhanced surveillance and early warning systems are essential for monitoring shifts in malaria transmission patterns and promptly identifying emerging hotspots. By leveraging advances in remote sensing, Geographic Information Systems (GIS), and modelling techniques, stakeholders can anticipate changes in vector distribution and prioritise resources for targeted interventions [78]. Community engagement and capacity-building initiatives also play a crucial role in fostering resilience to climate-related malaria risks, empowering local populations to implement preventive measures and respond effectively to outbreaks.

Climate change represents a formidable challenge to malaria control and prevention efforts, necessitating adaptive strategies to safeguard public health. By understanding the complex interactions between climatic factors, mosquito vectors, and human populations, stakeholders can develop proactive interventions tailored to the evolving risk landscape. Through integrated approaches that harness scientific innovation, community participation, and robust surveillance systems, we can reduce the effects of climate change on malaria transmission and advance towards a malaria-free future.

Climate Change and Disease Surveillance: The Case of Malaria

Climate change influences malaria transmission through several mechanisms:

1. ***Temperature***: Warmer temperatures can expand the geographical range of *Anopheles* mosquitoes to higher altitudes and latitudes. Increased temperatures

also shorten the development time of *Plasmodium* parasites within mosquitoes, potentially leading to higher transmission rates [12].

2. ***Rainfall and Humidity***: Changes in rainfall patterns affect mosquito breeding sites. Increased rainfall can create more habitats for mosquitoes, while prolonged dry spells can reduce their population [71].

3. ***Extreme Weather Events***: Floods and cyclones can disrupt healthcare infrastructure, increasing vulnerability to malaria outbreaks in affected regions.

These factors underscore the need for disease surveillance systems that can adapt to the evolving epidemiological landscape. Addressing the challenges posed by climate change to malaria control requires advancements in surveillance technology and methodologies. Several innovations have emerged to track and predict the spread of malaria more effectively:

1. ***Remote Sensing and Geographic Information Systems (GIS)***: Remote sensing technologies and GIS have revolutionized malaria surveillance. Satellite data can monitor environmental conditions, such as temperature, humidity, and vegetation, which influence mosquito habitats [12, 71, 79]. These technologies enable the creation of predictive models that forecast malaria outbreaks by correlating climatic data with disease incidence [78].

2. ***Climate-Based Predictive Modelling***: Advanced predictive models incorporate climate variables to forecast malaria risk. These models use machine learning algorithms to analyse large datasets, including historical climate data, mosquito population dynamics, and malaria case reports. By predicting potential outbreaks, these models inform targeted interventions, such as vector control measures and preemptive healthcare deployment [9].

3. ***Mobile Health (mHealth) Technologies***: mHealth applications enhance disease reporting and data collection, particularly in remote and resource-limited settings [80]. Health workers can use smartphones and tablets to report malaria cases in real-time, improving the speed and accuracy of surveillance. These tools also facilitate community engagement and education, which are crucial for effective malaria prevention and control [81].

4. ***Genomic Surveillance***: Genomic tools allow for the monitoring of mosquito and parasite populations at a genetic level. By sequencing the genomes of *Anopheles* mosquitoes and *Plasmodium* parasites, researchers can track the spread of drug-resistant strains and monitor changes in mosquito populations driven by climate change [16]. This information is vital for adapting treatment protocols and vector control strategies.

5. ***Integrated Disease Surveillance and Response (IDSR)***: The IDSR approach integrates data from various diseases and health conditions into a unified system, thereby enhancing the overall efficiency of public health surveillance [82]. By combining data on malaria with that on other climate-sensitive

diseases, health authorities can better allocate resources and respond to outbreaks more holistically.

Case Studies Highlighting the Successful Application of These Innovations

East Africa

In the highlands of East Africa, where malaria was previously uncommon, rising temperatures have led to increased transmission. Remote sensing data, combined with local health records, have been used to predict outbreaks, allowing for timely interventions, such as indoor residual spraying and the distribution of insecticide-treated nets [8, 9].

India

In Odisha, India, mHealth applications have been instrumental in reducing malaria incidence. Health workers equipped with mobile devices can report cases in real-time, enabling rapid response and resource allocation [83]. The integration of climate data into predictive models has further enhanced the effectiveness of these efforts.

Amazon Basin

Genomic surveillance in the Peruvian Amazon has provided insights into the spread of drug-resistant malaria [84]. By monitoring genetic mutations in *Plasmodium* parasites, researchers have adjusted treatment strategies and mitigated the impact of resistance.

Climate Policy and Health: Implications for Malaria Control

The intersection of climate policy and public health is increasingly critical as the global climate continues to change. One of the most significant impacts of climate change is its influence on the spread of infectious diseases, particularly vector-borne diseases, such as malaria. Environmental policies mitigating climate change can have direct and indirect effects on malaria control. These policies often involve strategies that alter land use, reduce greenhouse gas emissions, and promote renewable energy sources. Each of these strategies can influence malaria dynamics in different ways:

Land Use and Deforestation

Deforestation for agriculture or urban development can create new mosquito breeding sites by altering water drainage and increasing standing water [74].

Conversely, reforestation and sustainable land management can reduce malaria risk by stabilising ecosystems and reducing human exposure to mosquitoes.

Water Management

Policies promoting sustainable water use and the construction of valuable infrastructure, such as dams and irrigation systems, can impact mosquito breeding habitats. Properly managed water bodies can reduce mosquito breeding sites, whereas poorly managed ones can exacerbate the risk of malaria.

Urbanisation and Housing

Urban planning policies that ensure proper housing and sanitation can reduce human-mosquito contact. Improved housing with features such as screened windows and doors can significantly reduce malaria transmission rates.

Renewable Energy

Transitioning to renewable energy sources, such as solar, wind, and hydropower, reduces reliance on fossil fuels, thereby decreasing air pollution and mitigating climate change. Renewable energy projects can also enhance rural electrification, enabling better healthcare infrastructure and access to malaria prevention tools, including insecticide-treated nets and indoor residual spraying.

Carbon Sequestration

Efforts to increase carbon sequestration through afforestation and reforestation projects can contribute to ecosystem stability. Healthy forests can regulate local climates and water cycles, potentially reducing suitable habitats for malaria vectors.

Agricultural Practices

Climate-smart agriculture practices that enhance soil carbon storage and reduce emissions can also impact malaria control. Sustainable agriculture reduces the need for practices like slash-and-burn, which can create temporary mosquito habitats [74]. Moreover, crop diversification and integrated pest management can reduce mosquito breeding sites.

Integrating climate policy with health strategies is essential for effective malaria control in the face of climate change. Policymakers should consider the following approaches:

1. *Health Impact Assessments*: Conducting health impact assessments for major environmental policies ensures that potential health consequences, including malaria risks, are identified and addressed [85].
2. Intersectoral Collaboration: Collaboration among environmental, agricultural, and health sectors can lead to comprehensive strategies that simultaneously address climate mitigation and malaria control [73]. For example, coordinated efforts in water management can optimise irrigation practices to benefit both agricultural productivity and malaria prevention.
3. Community Engagement: Involving local communities in the planning and implementation of climate and health policies ensures that interventions are culturally appropriate and sustainable. Community-based monitoring and control programs can be effective in managing local malaria risks [86].
4. Research and Innovation: Continued research into the effects of climate change on malaria epidemiology is crucial. Innovations in vector control, such as the genetic modification of mosquitoes or the development of novel insecticides, can complement traditional methods and enhance resilience against climate-induced changes in malaria dynamics.

The intersection of climate policy and health, particularly in the context of malaria control, underscores the need for integrated and holistic approaches. Climate change mitigation strategies can have a profound impact on malaria transmission dynamics, necessitating careful consideration of both environmental and health outcomes. By aligning climate policies with public health goals, it is possible to create synergies that protect both the planet and human health, ultimately leading to more resilient and sustainable communities in the face of a changing climate.

Gradual Impact of Climate Change on Mosquito Habitats over Time

Climate change, a pressing global issue, manifests as alterations in temperatures, precipitation patterns, and extreme weather events [4, 5, 13, 14]. These environmental shifts have profound implications for ecosystems, including the habitats of mosquitoes, which are primary vectors of diseases such as malaria. Understanding the impact of climate change on mosquito habitats is crucial for predicting changes in disease transmission dynamics and implementing effective public health interventions.

Temperature is a critical factor in the lifecycle and distribution of mosquitoes [71]. Different mosquito species, including *Anopheles gambiae*, the primary vector for malaria in Africa, thrive within specific temperature ranges [12]. Generally, warmer temperatures accelerate mosquito development, enhance biting rates, and shorten the incubation period of the malaria parasite (*Plasmodium falciparum*) within the mosquito [87].

As global temperatures rise, the geographical range of mosquitoes is expanding. Warmer climates enable mosquitoes to inhabit higher altitudes and latitudes where they were previously unable to survive [88]. For instance, regions of East Africa, which were once too cool for malaria transmission, are now witnessing an increase in cases as mosquitoes colonise new areas [9, 30]. Similarly, parts of Europe and North America, which historically had minimal malaria risk, could become susceptible to outbreaks as conditions become more favourable for mosquitoes. However, extremely high temperatures can also be detrimental to mosquitoes. When temperatures exceed the optimal range for mosquito development (generally around 25-27°C for many species), mosquito survival rates can decline [89]. Thus, while some regions may see an increase in mosquito populations, others, particularly those already experiencing high temperatures, may witness a decline (Fig. 3).

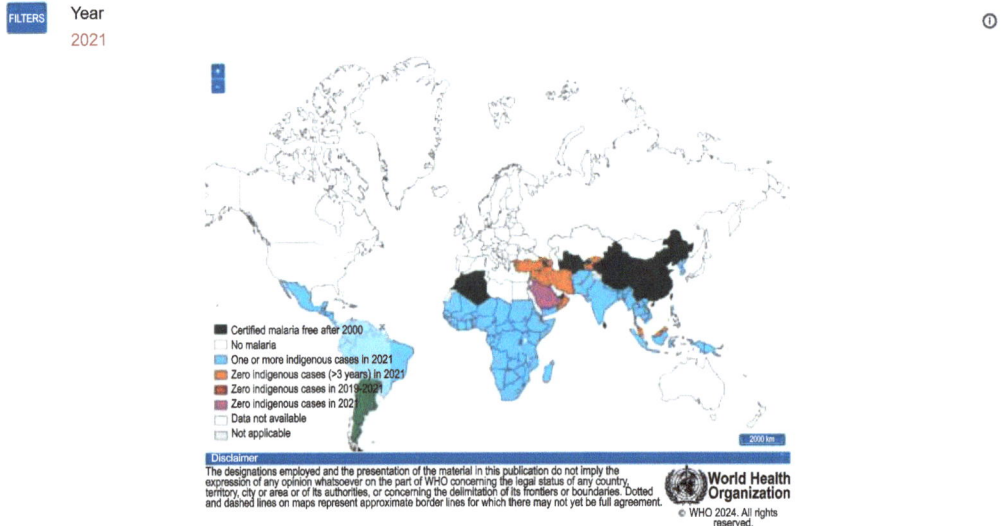

Status of indigenous malaria cases

FILTERS   Year
          2021

Certified malaria free after 2000
No malaria
One or more indigenous cases in 2021
Zero indigenous cases (>3 years) in 2021
Zero indigenous cases in 2019-2021
Zero indigenous cases in 2021
Data not available
Not applicable

Disclaimer
The designations employed and the presentation of the material in this publication do not imply the expression of any opinion whatsoever on the part of WHO concerning the legal status of any country, territory, city or area or of its authorities, or concerning the delimitation of its frontiers or boundaries. Dotted and dashed lines on maps represent approximate border lines for which there may not yet be full agreement.

World Health Organization
© WHO 2024. All rights reserved.

Fig. (3). Countries with zero indigenous malaria cases for three consecutive years are considered malaria-free. In 2021, Iran and Malaysia reported their fourth consecutive year with no cases, while Belize and Cabo Verde reported their third consecutive year. China and El Salvador were certified malaria-free in 2021 after four years without cases. *(Source: World malaria report 2022 - WHO).*

Precipitation significantly influences mosquito breeding sites [11]. Mosquitoes breed in stagnant or slow-moving water, making rainfall patterns a critical determinant of habitat availability. Climate change is altering these patterns, resulting in both increased and decreased rainfall in various regions. Increased rainfall can create abundant breeding sites, thereby boosting mosquito populations [11]. For example, regions experiencing heavier and more frequent rainfall may see an increase in the number of temporary water bodies, such as puddles and ditches, which are ideal for mosquito breeding. This can lead to higher mosquito densities and potentially more intense malaria transmission [11]. Conversely, regions experiencing decreased rainfall or prolonged dry spells may see a reduction in available breeding sites. However, this does not necessarily translate to reduced malaria transmission. In some cases, drought conditions can lead to the creation of artificial water storage solutions, such as water containers, which can become breeding grounds for mosquitoes. Additionally, stagnant water bodies that do not evaporate due to infrequent rainfall can become persistent mosquito habitats.

The combined effect of changing temperatures and precipitation patterns due to climate change significantly influences malaria transmission risk [11]. In regions where conditions become more favourable for mosquitoes, increased mosquito populations can lead to higher transmission rates of malaria. This is particularly concerning in areas with limited healthcare infrastructure and resources for mosquito control. Regions at the fringes of malaria-endemic areas are especially vulnerable. As mosquitoes expand their range, populations that previously had little exposure to malaria may face new risks. This can lead to higher morbidity and mortality rates, as these populations may lack immunity and access to effective treatment. Furthermore, climate change can influence the seasonality of malaria transmission. Warmer temperatures and altered precipitation can extend the transmission season in certain areas, resulting in a longer period of risk each year. This can strain public health systems and complicate efforts to control and prevent malaria.

Vector control measures, such as the use of Insecticide-treated Nets (ITNs), Indoor Residual Spraying (IRS), and environmental management to reduce breeding sites, remain critical [8]. However, considering the evolving environmental conditions, these interventions must be tailored to the local context. Additionally, integrating climate information into public health planning can improve the predictability and effectiveness of interventions. Climate models that forecast temperature and precipitation changes can help anticipate shifts in mosquito habitats and inform proactive measures.

Climate change profoundly impacts mosquito habitats through alterations in temperature and precipitation patterns, influencing the risk of malaria transmission [11]. As global temperatures continue to rise and precipitation patterns shift, adaptive and advanced approaches will be crucial in protecting vulnerable populations and preventing the resurgence of malaria in new regions.

CONCLUSION

Climate change presents a formidable challenge to malaria control, but it also spurs innovation in disease surveillance and prediction. By harnessing remote sensing, predictive modelling, mHealth, genomic tools, and integrated surveillance systems, public health authorities can better anticipate and respond to malaria outbreaks. Continued investment in these technologies and international cooperation will be crucial to protecting vulnerable populations and achieving long-term malaria control in a changing climate.

These topics can provide a multidimensional view of the intersection between climate change and malaria, offering insights into both the direct and indirect effects of environmental changes on malaria transmission. They also facilitate an in-depth investigation into the broader implications of this intersection on public health, policy, and global efforts to combat climate change and its impact on this disease.

REFERENCES

[1]   Fikadu M, Ashenafi E. Malaria: An Overview. Infect Drug Resist 2023; 16: 3339-47.
       [http://dx.doi.org/10.2147/IDR.S405668] [PMID: 37274361]

[2]   Abouelfadl S. Global warming - causes, effects and solution's trials. JES Journal of Engineering Sciences 2012; 40(4): 1233-54.
       [http://dx.doi.org/10.21608/jesaun.2012.114490]

[3]   Rohr JR, Dobson AP, Johnson PTJ, *et al.* Frontiers in climate change–disease research. Trends Ecol Evol 2011; 26(6): 270-7.
       [http://dx.doi.org/10.1016/j.tree.2011.03.002] [PMID: 21481487]

[4]   Carvalho BM, Rangel EF, Vale MM. Evaluation of the impacts of climate change on disease vectors through ecological niche modelling. Bull Entomol Res 2017; 107(4): 419-30.
       [http://dx.doi.org/10.1017/S0007485316001097] [PMID: 27974065]

[5]   Jia P, Chen X, Chen J, Lu L, Liu Q, Tan X. How does the dengue vector mosquito *Aedes albopictus* respond to global warming? Parasit Vectors 2017; 10(1): 140.
       [http://dx.doi.org/10.1186/s13071-017-2071-2] [PMID: 28284225]

[6]   Tonnang HEZ, Kangalawe RYM, Yanda PZ. Predicting and mapping malaria under climate change scenarios: the potential redistribution of malaria vectors in Africa. Malar J 2010; 9(1): 111.
       [http://dx.doi.org/10.1186/1475-2875-9-111] [PMID: 20416059]

[7]   Asad H, Carpenter DO. Effects of climate change on the spread of zika virus: a public health threat. Rev Environ Health 2018; 33(1): 31-42.
       [http://dx.doi.org/10.1515/reveh-2017-0042] [PMID: 29500926]

[8]   Benelli G, Beier JC. Current vector control challenges in the fight against malaria. Acta Trop 2017; 174: 91-6.
       [http://dx.doi.org/10.1016/j.actatropica.2017.06.028] [PMID: 28684267]

[9]   Githeko AK, Ogallo L, Lemnge M, Okia M, Ototo EN. Development and validation of climate and ecosystem-based early malaria epidemic prediction models in East Africa. Malar J 2014; 13(1): 329.
       [http://dx.doi.org/10.1186/1475-2875-13-329] [PMID: 25149479]

[10]   Kripa PK, Thanzeen PS, Jaganathasamy N, Ravishankaran S, Anvikar AR, Eapen A. Impact of climate

change on temperature variations and extrinsic incubation period of malaria parasites in Chennai, India: implications for its disease transmission potential. Parasit Vectors 2024; 17(1): 134.
[http://dx.doi.org/10.1186/s13071-024-06165-0] [PMID: 38491547]

[11] Stresman GH. Beyond temperature and precipitation: Ecological risk factors that modify malaria transmission. Acta Trop 2010; 116(3): 167-72.
[http://dx.doi.org/10.1016/j.actatropica.2010.08.005] [PMID: 20727338]

[12] Beck-Johnson LM, Nelson WA, Paaijmans KP, Read AF, Thomas MB, Bjørnstad ON. The effect of temperature on *Anopheles* mosquito population dynamics and the potential for malaria transmission. PLoS One 2013; 8(11): e79276.
[http://dx.doi.org/10.1371/journal.pone.0079276] [PMID: 24244467]

[13] Sáenz R, Bissell RA, Paniagua F. Post-disaster malaria in costa rica. Prehosp Disaster Med 1995; 10(3): 154-60.
[http://dx.doi.org/10.1017/S1049023X00041935] [PMID: 10155423]

[14] Mason J, Cavalie P. Malaria epidemic in haiti following a hurricane. Am J Trop Med Hyg 1965; 14(4): 533-9.
[http://dx.doi.org/10.4269/ajtmh.1965.14.533]

[15] Haldar K, Bhattacharjee S, Safeukui I. Drug resistance in *plasmodium*. Nat Rev Microbiol 2018; 16(3): 156-70.
[http://dx.doi.org/10.1038/nrmicro.2017.161] [PMID: 29355852]

[16] Nsanzabana C, Djalle D, Guérin PJ, Ménard D, González IJ. Tools for surveillance of anti-malarial drug resistance: an assessment of the current landscape. Malar J 2018; 17(1): 75.
[http://dx.doi.org/10.1186/s12936-018-2185-9] [PMID: 29422048]

[17] Malaria S. Severe Malaria. Trop Med Int Health 2014; 19(s1) (Suppl. 1): 7-131.
[http://dx.doi.org/10.1111/tmi.12313_2] [PMID: 25214480]

[18] Clements AN. Biology of mosquitoes: Development nutrition and reproduction. Springer 1992.
[http://dx.doi.org/10.1079/9780851993744.0000]

[19] Breman JG, Egan A, Keusch GT. The intolerable burden of malaria: a new look at the numbers. Am J Trop Med Hyg 2001; 64(1_Suppl) (Suppl.): iv-vii.
[http://dx.doi.org/10.4269/ajtmh.2001.64.iv] [PMID: 11425185]

[20] Snow RW, Craig M, Deichmann U, Marsh K. Estimating mortality, morbidity and disability due to malaria among Africa's non-pregnant population. Bull World Health Organ 1999; 77(8): 624-40.
[PMID: 10516785]

[21] Tuteja R. Malaria – an overview. FEBS J 2007; 274(18): 4670-9.
[http://dx.doi.org/10.1111/j.1742-4658.2007.05997.x] [PMID: 17824953]

[22] Cox Feg. History of the discovery of the malaria parasites and their vectors. Parasit Vectors 2010; 3(1): 5.
[http://dx.doi.org/10.1186/1756-3305-3-5] [PMID: 20205846]

[23] Dagen M. History of malaria and its treatment Antimalarial Agents. Elsevier 2020; pp. 1-48.
[http://dx.doi.org/10.1016/B978-0-08-101210-9.00001-9]

[24] Korenromp E. Malaria incidence estimates at country level for the year 2004 Proposed estimates and draft report.

[25] Hay SI, Guerra CA, Tatem AJ, Noor AM, Snow RW. The global distribution and population at risk of malaria: past, present, and future. Lancet Infect Dis 2004; 4(6): 327-36.
[http://dx.doi.org/10.1016/S1473-3099(04)01043-6] [PMID: 15172341]

[26] Murray CJL, Rosenfeld LC, Lim SS, *et al.* Global malaria mortality between 1980 and 2010: a systematic analysis. Lancet 2012; 379(9814): 413-31.
[http://dx.doi.org/10.1016/S0140-6736(12)60034-8] [PMID: 22305225]

[27] Guinovart C, Navia M, Tanner M, Alonso P. Malaria: Burden of Disease. Curr Mol Med 2006; 6(2): 137-40.
[http://dx.doi.org/10.2174/156652406776055131] [PMID: 16515506]

[28] Al-Awadhi M, Ahmad S, Iqbal J. Current status and the epidemiology of malaria in the middle east region and beyond. Microorganisms 2021; 9(2): 338.
[http://dx.doi.org/10.3390/microorganisms9020338] [PMID: 33572053]

[29] Sinka ME, Bangs MJ, Manguin S, *et al.* The dominant *Anopheles* vectors of human malaria in the Asia-Pacific region: occurrence data, distribution maps and bionomic précis. Parasit Vectors 2011; 4(1): 89.
[http://dx.doi.org/10.1186/1756-3305-4-89] [PMID: 21612587]

[30] Sinka ME, Pironon S, Massey NC, *et al.* A new malaria vector in Africa: Predicting the expansion range of *Anopheles stephensi* and identifying the urban populations at risk. Proc Natl Acad Sci USA 2020; 117(40): 24900-8.
[http://dx.doi.org/10.1073/pnas.2003976117] [PMID: 32929020]

[31] Ahmed A, Pignatelli P, Elaagip A, Abdel Hamid MM, Alrahman OF, Weetman D. Invasive malaria vector *anopheles stephensi* mosquitoes in sudan, 2016–2018. Emerg Infect Dis 2021; 27(11): 2952-4.
[http://dx.doi.org/10.3201/eid2711.210040] [PMID: 34670658]

[32] Hamlet A, Dengela D, Tongren JE, *et al.* The potential impact of *Anopheles stephensi* establishment on the transmission of *Plasmodium falciparum* in Ethiopia and prospective control measures. BMC Med 2022; 20(1): 135.
[http://dx.doi.org/10.1186/s12916-022-02324-1] [PMID: 35440085]

[33] Subbarao SK, Vasantha K, Adak T, Sharma VP, Curtis CF. Egg-float ridge number in *Anopheles stephensi*: ecological variation and genetic analysis. Med Vet Entomol 1987; 1(3): 265-71.
[http://dx.doi.org/10.1111/j.1365-2915.1987.tb00353.x] [PMID: 2979540]

[34] Thomas S, Ravishankaran S, Justin NAJA, *et al.* Resting and feeding preferences of *Anopheles stephensi* in an urban setting, perennial for malaria. Malar J 2017; 16(1): 111.
[http://dx.doi.org/10.1186/s12936-017-1764-5] [PMID: 28283033]

[35] Knols BGJ. Review of "Mosquitoes of the World" by Richard C. Wilkerson, Yvonne-Marie Linton, and Daniel Strickman. Parasit Vectors 2021; 14(1): 341.
[http://dx.doi.org/10.1186/s13071-021-04848-6]

[36] Wheelwright M, Whittle CR, Riabinina O. Olfactory systems across mosquito species. Cell Tissue Res 2021; 383(1): 75-90.
[http://dx.doi.org/10.1007/s00441-020-03407-2] [PMID: 33475852]

[37] Weiss DJ, Lucas TCD, Nguyen M, *et al.* Mapping the global prevalence, incidence, and mortality of *Plasmodium falciparum*, 2000–17: a spatial and temporal modelling study. Lancet 2019; 394(10195): 322-31.
[http://dx.doi.org/10.1016/S0140-6736(19)31097-9] [PMID: 31229234]

[38] Hinton HE. Observations on the biology and taxonomy of the eggs of *Anopheles* mosquitos. Bull Entomol Res 1968; 57(4): 495-508.
[http://dx.doi.org/10.1017/S0007485300052858] [PMID: 5659158]

[39] Malhotra PR, Jatav PC, Chauhan RS. Surface morphology of the egg of *Anopheles stephensi* sensu stricto (*diptera, culicidae*). Ital J Zool (Modena) 2000; 67(2): 147-51.
[http://dx.doi.org/10.1080/11250000009356307]

[40] Nathan D. Burkett-Cadena Mosquitoes of the southeastern United States. University of Alabama Press 2013.

[41] Foster WA, Walker ED. Mosquitoes (Culicidae) Med Vet Entomol. Elsevier 2019; pp. 261-325.
[http://dx.doi.org/10.1016/B978-0-12-814043-7.00015-7]

[42]   Manda H, Gouagna LC, Foster WA, *et al.* Effect of discriminative plant-sugar feeding on the survival and fecundity of *Anopheles gambiae*. Malar J 2007; 6(1): 113.
[http://dx.doi.org/10.1186/1475-2875-6-113] [PMID: 17711580]

[43]   Smith GE, Watson RB, Crowell RL. Observations on the flight range of *anopheles quadrimaculatus*, say. Am J Hyg 1942; 34: 102-13.

[44]   Guerin PJ, Olliaro P, Nosten F, *et al.* Malaria: current status of control, diagnosis, treatment, and a proposed agenda for research and development. Lancet Infect Dis 2002; 2(9): 564-73.
[http://dx.doi.org/10.1016/S1473-3099(02)00372-9] [PMID: 12206972]

[45]   Moyes CL, Henry AJ, Golding N, *et al.* Defining the geographical range of the *Plasmodium knowlesi* reservoir. PLoS Negl Trop Dis 2014; 8(3): e2780.
[http://dx.doi.org/10.1371/journal.pntd.0002780] [PMID: 24676231]

[46]   Rodríguez-Morales AJ, Sánchez E, Vargas M, *et al.* Is anemia in *Plasmodium vivax* malaria more frequent and severe than in *Plasmodium falciparum*? Am J Med 2006; 119(11): e9-e10.
[http://dx.doi.org/10.1016/j.amjmed.2005.08.014] [PMID: 17071151]

[47]   Robinson LJ, Wampfler R, Betuela I, *et al.* Strategies for understanding and reducing the *Plasmodium vivax* and *Plasmodium ovale* hypnozoite reservoir in Papua New Guinean children: a randomised placebo-controlled trial and mathematical model. PLoS Med 2015; 12(10): e1001891.
[http://dx.doi.org/10.1371/journal.pmed.1001891] [PMID: 26505753]

[48]   Beier JC. Malaria parasite development in mosquitoes. Annu Rev Entomol 1998; 43(1): 519-43.
[http://dx.doi.org/10.1146/annurev.ento.43.1.519] [PMID: 9444756]

[49]   Baer K, Klotz C, Kappe SHI, Schnieder T, Frevert U. Release of hepatic *Plasmodium yoelii* merozoites into the pulmonary microvasculature. PLoS Pathog 2007; 3(11): e171.
[http://dx.doi.org/10.1371/journal.ppat.0030171] [PMID: 17997605]

[50]   Frevert U, Krzych U. *Plasmodium* cellular effector mechanisms and the hepatic microenvironment. Front Microbiol 2015; 6: 482.
[http://dx.doi.org/10.3389/fmicb.2015.00482] [PMID: 26074888]

[51]   Burda PC, Caldelari R, Heussler VT. Manipulation of the host cell membrane during *Plasmodium* liver stage egress. MBio 2017; 8(2): e00139-17.
[http://dx.doi.org/10.1128/mBio.00139-17] [PMID: 28400525]

[52]   Collins WE, Jeffery GM. *Plasmodium malariae* : Parasite and Disease. Clin Microbiol Rev 2007; 20(4): 579-92.
[http://dx.doi.org/10.1128/CMR.00027-07] [PMID: 17934075]

[53]   Xie SC, Dogovski C, Hanssen E, Chiu F, Yang T, Crespo MP. Haemoglobin degradation underpins the sensitivity of early ring stage *Plasmodium falciparum* to artemisinins. J Cell Sci 2015; .
[http://dx.doi.org/10.1242/jcs.178830] [PMID: 26675237]

[54]   Cowman AF, Crabb BS. The *Plasmodium falciparum* genome--a blueprint for erythrocyte invasion. Science 2002; 298(5591): 126-8.
[http://dx.doi.org/10.1126/science.1078169] [PMID: 12364790]

[55]   Tran TM, Moreno A, Yazdani SS, Chitnis CE, Barnwell JW, Galinski MR. Detection of a *Plasmodium vivax* erythrocyte binding protein by flow cytometry. Cytometry A 2005; 63A(1): 59-66.
[http://dx.doi.org/10.1002/cyto.a.20098] [PMID: 15584018]

[56]   Kraemer SM, Smith JD. A family affair: var genes, PfEMP1 binding, and malaria disease. Curr Opin Microbiol 2006; 9(4): 374-80.
[http://dx.doi.org/10.1016/j.mib.2006.06.006] [PMID: 16814594]

[57]   Amit-Avraham I, Pozner G, Eshar S, Fastman Y, Kolevzon N, Yavin E, *et al.* Antisense long noncoding RNAs regulate *var* gene activation in the malaria parasite *Plasmodium falciparum*. Proceedings of the National Academy of Sciences.

[http://dx.doi.org/10.1073/pnas.1420855112]

[58]   Chookajorn T, Dzikowski R, Frank M, *et al.* Epigenetic memory at malaria virulence genes. Proc Natl Acad Sci USA 2007; 104(3): 899-902.
[http://dx.doi.org/10.1073/pnas.0609084103] [PMID: 17209011]

[59]   Beeson JG, Brown GV, Molyneux ME, Mhango C, Dzinjalamala F, Rogerson SJ. *Plasmodium falciparum* isolates from infected pregnant women and children are associated with distinct adhesive and antigenic properties. J Infect Dis 1999; 180(2): 464-72.
[http://dx.doi.org/10.1086/314899] [PMID: 10395863]

[60]   Eksi S, Czesny B, Van Gemert GJ, Sauerwein RW, Eling W, Williamson KC. Malaria transmission-blocking antigen, Pfs230, mediates human red blood cell binding to exflagellating male parasites and oocyst production. Mol Microbiol 2006; 61(4): 991-8.
[http://dx.doi.org/10.1111/j.1365-2958.2006.05284.x] [PMID: 16879650]

[61]   Baruch DI. Adhesive receptors on malaria-parasitized red cells. Best Pract Res Clin Haematol 1999; 12(4): 747-61.
[http://dx.doi.org/10.1053/beha.1999.0051] [PMID: 10895262]

[62]   Ockenhouse CF, Ho M, Tandon NN, *et al.* Molecular basis of sequestration in severe and uncomplicated Plasmodium falciparum malaria: differential adhesion of infected erythrocytes to CD36 and ICAM-1. J Infect Dis 1991; 164(1): 163-9.
[http://dx.doi.org/10.1093/infdis/164.1.163] [PMID: 1711552]

[63]   Newbold C, Craig A, Kyes S, Rowe A, Fernandez-Reyes D, Fagan T. Cytoadherence, pathogenesis and the infected red cell surface in *Plasmodium falciparum*. Int J Parasitol 1999; 29(6): 927-37.
[http://dx.doi.org/10.1016/S0020-7519(99)00049-1] [PMID: 10480730]

[64]   Miller LH, Baruch DI, Marsh K, Doumbo OK. The pathogenic basis of malaria. Nature 2002; 415(6872): 673-9.
[http://dx.doi.org/10.1038/415673a] [PMID: 11832955]

[65]   Snow RW, Marsh K. New insights into the epidemiology of malaria relevant for disease control. Br Med Bull 1998; 54(2): 293-309.
[http://dx.doi.org/10.1093/oxfordjournals.bmb.a011689] [PMID: 9830198]

[66]   Bell D, Wongsrichanalai C, Barnwell JW. Ensuring quality and access for malaria diagnosis: how can it be achieved? Nat Rev Microbiol 2006; 4(9): 682-95.
[http://dx.doi.org/10.1038/nrmicro1474] [PMID: 16912713]

[67]   Bell D, Wongsrichanalai C, Barnwell JW. Ensuring quality and access for malaria diagnosis: how can it be achieved? Nat Rev Microbiol 2006; 4(9): 682-95.
[http://dx.doi.org/10.1038/nrmicro1474] [PMID: 16912713]

[68]   Ridley RG. Medical need, scientific opportunity and the drive for antimalarial drugs. Nature 2002; 415(6872): 686-93.
[http://dx.doi.org/10.1038/415686a] [PMID: 11832957]

[69]   Heddini A, Gerald T. Keusch, Catherine S. Davies. The multilateral initiative on malaria: past, present, and future. Am J Trop Med Hyg 2004; 71.
[http://dx.doi.org/DOI:10.4269/ajtmh.2004.71.279]

[70]   Marrelli MT, Li C, Rasgon JL, Jacobs-Lorena M. Transgenic malaria-resistant mosquitoes have a fitness advantage when feeding on *Plasmodium* -infected blood. Proc Natl Acad Sci USA 2007; 104(13): 5580-3.
[http://dx.doi.org/10.1073/pnas.0609809104] [PMID: 17372227]

[71]   Liu Z, Wang S, Zhang Y, *et al.* Effect of temperature and its interactions with relative humidity and rainfall on malaria in a temperate city Suzhou, China. Environ Sci Pollut Res Int 2021; 28(13): 16830-42.
[http://dx.doi.org/10.1007/s11356-020-12138-4] [PMID: 33394450]

[72] Shretta R, Avanceña ALV, Hatefi A. The economics of malaria control and elimination: a systematic review. Malar J 2016; 15(1): 593.
[http://dx.doi.org/10.1186/s12936-016-1635-5] [PMID: 27955665]

[73] Naing C, Whittaker MA, Tanner M. Inter-sectoral approaches for the prevention and control of malaria among the mobile and migrant populations: a scoping review. Malar J 2018; 17(1): 430.
[http://dx.doi.org/10.1186/s12936-018-2562-4] [PMID: 30445959]

[74] Asenso-Okyere K, Asante FA, Tarekegn J, Andam KS. A review of the economic impact of malaria in agricultural development. Agric Econ 2011; 42(3): 293-304.
[http://dx.doi.org/10.1111/j.1574-0862.2010.00515.x]

[75] Laurens MB. RTS,S/AS01 vaccine (Mosquirix™): an overview. Hum Vaccin Immunother 2020; 16(3): 480-9.
[http://dx.doi.org/10.1080/21645515.2019.1669415] [PMID: 31545128]

[76] Datoo MS, Natama HM, Somé A, *et al.* Efficacy and immunogenicity of R21/Matrix-M vaccine against clinical malaria after 2 years' follow-up in children in Burkina Faso: a phase 1/2b randomised controlled trial. Lancet Infect Dis 2022; 22(12): 1728-36.
[http://dx.doi.org/10.1016/S1473-3099(22)00442-X] [PMID: 36087586]

[77] Efficacy and safety of RTS,S/AS01 malaria vaccine with or without a booster dose in infants and children in Africa: final results of a phase 3, individually randomised, controlled trial. Lancet 2015; 386(9988): 31-45.
[http://dx.doi.org/10.1016/S0140-6736(15)60721-8] [PMID: 25913272]

[78] Palaniyandi M. The role of remote sensing and gis for spatial prediction of vector-borne diseases transmission: A systematic review. J Vector Borne Dis 2012; 49(4): 197-204.
[http://dx.doi.org/10.4103/0972-9062.213498] [PMID: 23428518]

[79] Nik Abdull Halim NMH, Che Dom N, Dapari R, Salim H, Precha N. A systematic review and meta-analysis of the effects of temperature on the development and survival of the *Aedes* mosquito. Front Public Health 2022; 10: 1074028.
[http://dx.doi.org/10.3389/fpubh.2022.1074028] [PMID: 36600940]

[80] Larocca A, Moro Visconti R, Marconi M. Malaria diagnosis and mapping with m-Health and Geographic Information Systems (GIS): evidence from Uganda. Malar J 2016; 15(1): 520.
[http://dx.doi.org/10.1186/s12936-016-1546-5] [PMID: 27776516]

[81] Mangam K, Fiekowsky E, Bagayoko M, *et al.* Feasibility and effectiveness of health for mobilizing households for indoor residual spraying to prevent malaria: A case study in mali. Glob Health Sci Pract 2016; 4(2): 222-37.
[http://dx.doi.org/10.9745/GHSP-D-15-00381] [PMID: 27353616]

[82] Wolfe CM, Hamblion EL, Dzotsi EK, *et al.* Systematic review of Integrated Disease Surveillance and Response (IDSR) implementation in the African region. PLoS One 2021; 16(2): e0245457.
[http://dx.doi.org/10.1371/journal.pone.0245457] [PMID: 33630890]

[83] Majumdar A. mHealth in the prevention and control of non-communicable diseases in India: current possibilities and the way forward. J Clin Diagn Res 2015.
[http://dx.doi.org/10.7860/JCDR/2015/11555.5573]

[84] Cowell AN, Valdivia HO, Bishop DK, Winzeler EA. Exploration of *Plasmodium vivax* transmission dynamics and recurrent infections in the Peruvian Amazon using whole genome sequencing. Genome Med 2018; 10(1): 52.
[http://dx.doi.org/10.1186/s13073-018-0563-0] [PMID: 29973248]

[85] Rowe AK. Assessing the health impact of malaria control interventions in the MDG/sustainable development goal Era: A new generation of impact evaluations. Am J Trop Med Hyg 2017; 97(3_Suppl): 6-8.
[http://dx.doi.org/10.4269/ajtmh.17-0509] [PMID: 28990917]

[86]   Whittaker M, Smith C. Reimagining malaria: five reasons to strengthen community engagement in the lead up to malaria elimination. Malar J 2015; 14(1): 410.
[http://dx.doi.org/10.1186/s12936-015-0931-9] [PMID: 26474852]

[87]   Agyekum TP, Botwe PK, Arko-Mensah J, *et al.* A systematic review of the effects of temperature on *Anopheles* mosquito development and survival: Implications for malaria control in a future warmer climate. Int J Environ Res Public Health 2021; 18(14): 7255.
[http://dx.doi.org/10.3390/ijerph18147255] [PMID: 34299706]

[88]   Lozano-Fuentes S, Hayden MH, Welsh-Rodriguez C, *et al.* The dengue virus mosquito vector *Aedes aegypti* at high elevation in Mexico. Am J Trop Med Hyg 2012; 87(5): 902-9.
[http://dx.doi.org/10.4269/ajtmh.2012.12-0244] [PMID: 22987656]

[89]   Reinhold J, Lazzari C, Lahondère C. Effects of the environmental temperature on *Aedes aegypti* and *Aedes albopictus* mosquitoes: A review. Insects 2018; 9(4): 158.
[http://dx.doi.org/10.3390/insects9040158] [PMID: 30404142]

CHAPTER 6

Climate Change and Crimean-Congo Hemorrhagic Fever (CCHF)

R Narendar[1] and **Jayalakshmi Krishnan[1,*]**

[1] *Vector Biology Research Laboratory, Department of Biotechnology, Central University of Tamil Nadu, Thiruvarur, India*

Abstract: Crimean-Congo Hemorrhagic Fever (CCHF) is a highly virulent viral disease characterized by a rapid onset of symptoms and significant mortality rates. The primary mode of transmission to humans is through tick bites, particularly from the *Hyalomma* genus, or through direct contact with infected animals or humans. Clinically, CCHF typically begins with the abrupt onset of fever, myalgia, headache, nausea, vomiting, and diarrhea. As the disease advances, patients may exhibit severe hemorrhagic manifestations, including extensive bruising, epistaxis, and uncontrolled bleeding from venipuncture sites. The progression can result in multi-organ failure, with a fatality rate of up to 40%. CCHF is endemic in regions of Africa, Asia, Eastern Europe, and the Mediterranean. Recent decades have seen an expansion of its geographic range, attributed to factors such as climate change and increased global movement. Populations at elevated risk include healthcare workers and individuals involved in livestock handling and meat processing. Currently, the management of CCHF is primarily supportive, as there are no specific antiviral treatments approved for this disease. Key preventive measures include avoiding tick bites, adhering to safe practices during meat processing, and using personal protective equipment properly. Continuous surveillance, ongoing research, and robust public health preparedness are crucial to address this escalating global health threat effectively.

Keywords: CCHFV, Climate changes, Crimean-Congo Hemorrhagic Fever, Infection control, Nairovirus, Public health, Ribavirin, Tick-borne disease, Vaccine development, Viral hemorrhagic fever.

INTRODUCTION

Crimean-Congo Hemorrhagic Fever (CCHF) is a highly virulent viral disease characterized by its swift transmission and severe clinical symptoms. Historically prevalent in Africa, Asia, and Eastern Europe, CCHF has emerged as a global health concern, drawing significant attention from the scientific and medical

* **Corresponding author Jayalakshmi Krishnan:** Vector Biology Research Laboratory, Department of Biotechnology, Central University of Tamil Nadu, Thiruvarur, India; E-mail: jayalakshmi@cutn.ac.in

Jayalakshmi Krishnan, Sigamani Panneer, P. Thiyagarajan, Balachandar Vellingiri & Pradeep Kumar Srivastava (Eds.)

communities [1]. Upon infection, CCHF initially presents with flu-like symptoms, including high fever, severe headache, muscle pain, and malaise. Patients may experience gastrointestinal symptoms, such as nausea, vomiting, and diarrhea, as the disease progresses. Notably, hemorrhage is a hallmark feature of CCHF, leading to petechiae, ecchymosis, epistaxis, gingival bleeding, and gastrointestinal bleeding, highlighting the disease's severity and potential for devastating outcomes [2]. In severe cases, CCHF can cause organ dysfunction, including liver and kidney failure, ultimately resulting in death. The fatality rate of CCHF ranges from 10% to 30%, influenced by factors such as the virus strain and the availability of medical care. Despite advances in supportive care, specific antiviral treatments for CCHF are lacking, emphasizing the importance of preventive measures and early intervention strategies [1, 3]. CCHF is mainly transmitted to humans through the bite of infected ticks, especially those from the *Hyalomma* genus, which act as vectors and reservoirs for the virus. Healthcare workers and individuals engaged in animal husbandry, slaughter, or veterinary practices face substantial risks when they come into direct contact with the blood or bodily fluids of infected individuals. Additionally, occasional reports of aerosol transmission have been documented in healthcare settings and laboratory environments [3, 4].

The historical range of CCHF reflects the distribution of its primary vector, *Hyalomma* ticks, which thrive in warm climates and suitable habitats. The expansion of globalization and the effects of climate change have facilitated the transmission of CCHF into previously unaffected areas, highlighting the evolving landscape of infectious disease epidemiology and emphasizing the need for continuous monitoring and management of emerging risks, such as CCHF [5].

Crimean-Congo Hemorrhagic Fever [CCHF] is a significant and growing global health threat characterized by an increase in its geographic range and incidence in the 21st century [6]. The CCHF Virus [CCHFV] is responsible for the disease. It is primarily transmitted *via* ticks, posing a significant threat of multiple outbreaks, particularly in regions across Africa, Asia, the Middle East, and certain parts of Europe [2, 5].

Scientists first described Crimean-Congo Hemorrhagic Fever in the 20th century, but the disease likely affected people long before it was recognized. Crimean-Congo Hemorrhagic Fever is a potentially fatal virus initially spotted in the Crimean region during the 1940s [7]. Later, they identified it as the same pathogen responsible for what was once known as Congo Hemorrhagic Fever. The detection of the CCHF virus in regions of ancient Celtic settlements in Germany suggests its presence dating back to antiquity [8].

Known for being the most significant human disease spread by ticks, CCHF has affected people from western China to the Middle East, southeastern Europe, and throughout Africa. Over the last two decades, the disease has emerged in multiple locations, including Eastern Europe, particularly in post-Soviet states, the Mediterranean, Central Asia, Southern Europe, Africa, the Middle East, and the Indian subcontinent [1, 7].

Greece reported its first CCHF case in 2008, which resulted in the death of a woman. The disease has a long-standing presence in regions such as Africa, the Balkans, and South Asian countries below the 50th parallel north, which marks the habitat boundary for its primary carrier, the tick [9].

Transmission typically occurs through the bite of an infected tick or exposure to bodily fluids from an infected person or animal [7]. In various outbreaks, the fatality rate for CCHF among those hospitalized has varied widely, from as low as 9% to as high as 70%. However, the World Health Organization notes that it generally falls between 10% and 40% [10].

No commercial vaccines or specific approved treatments are available for CCHF, and care for those affected mostly involves supportive measures. Although neither the FDA nor the WHO has officially sanctioned it, some have suggested that the antiviral ribavirin may be beneficial [11]. Various factors contribute to the emergence and re-emergence of Crimean-Congo Hemorrhagic Fever [CCHF] in new regions.

Climate change and landscape transformations have impacted the abundance and spatial distribution of CCHFV animal hosts and vectors, significantly influencing transmission dynamics and increasing the likelihood of disease emergence [12]. Environmental changes, such as those seen in Turkey, have led to shifts in small mammal communities, resulting in the spillover of CCHF into human populations [13]. The Eastern Mediterranean Region has seen an emergence or re-emergence of CCHF in several countries over the last decade, with an increasing risk of extension into new areas. CCHF is increasingly recognized by the World Health Organization [WHO] as a significant and escalating health concern in the Eastern Mediterranean Region, as evidenced by new regions reporting cases and the disease spreading geographically. While strict adherence to infection control measures is essential for containing healthcare-associated outbreaks, these protocols are only sometimes followed, even in advanced settings [14].

In summary, CCHF poses an escalating global health risk due to its expanding geographic range, increasing incidence, and potential for outbreaks driven by environmental changes and inadequate infection control practices. Continued surveillance, research, and public health preparedness are necessary to address this emerging threat.

Climate change significantly contributes to the spread of Crimean-Congo Hemorrhagic Fever [CCHF] into new regions. Changing temperatures and shifting precipitation patterns modify the environments where ticks reside, including the hard-bodied *Hyalomma marginatum* ticks that carry the CCHF virus [5, 12]. These environmental changes enable the ticks to thrive in areas that were previously unsuitable for them. For instance, climate change has facilitated the northward movement of these ticks through Europe, leading to the first reported cases of CCHF in Spain in 2011 and 2016. In Turkey, environmental changes have shifted small mammal populations, leading to an increased spillover of CCHF into human populations. Over the past decade, CCHF has emerged or re-emerged in multiple countries within the Eastern Mediterranean Region, with the disease expanding into new areas [13, 14]. The World Health Organization [WHO] has recognized CCHF as a growing health threat in this region, noting that new areas report cases, indicating a geographic expansion of the disease [15]. Factors such as climate change, changes in land use, recreational activities, and the trade of infected animals are likely to make this deadly disease more common. Consequently, the expanding geographic range and increasing incidence of CCHF, attributed to climate change, pose a serious and growing global health threat. Ongoing surveillance, research, and public health preparedness are crucial for addressing this emerging infectious disease [16].

CCHF

The Crimean-Congo hemorrhagic fever virus is transmitted by ticks that belong to the genus Orthonairovirus, part of the Nairoviridae family, within the order Bunyavirales. As an enveloped virus that harbors a negative-sense RNA genome divided into three segments labeled Small [S], Medium [M], and Large [L], it exhibits a complex molecular structure. The S segment is responsible for coding the nucleocapsid protein, the M segment for the envelope glycoproteins Gc and Gn, which facilitate cell entry, and the L segment encodes both the RNA polymerase and an ovarian tumor protease domain [14 - 16].

Understanding the Virus at a Molecular Level

CCHFV's genetic material comprises three RNA segments enveloped by a surrounding layer of protein called the nucleoprotein, which is tightly associated with the RNA-dependent RNA polymerase protein, the L protein. These segments dictate the structure of the vital viral proteins, including the outer glycoproteins Gn and Gc, which play crucial roles in binding to receptors on a host cell to initiate infection [17].

Detailed Virology

Visually, the virus particles range in diameter from 80 to 120 nanometers, displaying a variable or pleomorphic shape. They encompass a trio of RNA strings that collectively form the viral genome [18]. The virus is encased in a monolayer lipid envelope approximately 5 nm thick, with proteins on this layer forming surface projections that are approximately 5–10 nm long. The extended, filamentous arrangements shape the internal nucleocapsids. Entry into host cells involves clathrin—a cellular protein—and may be associated with another cell surface component known as nucleolin [18, 19].

Patterns of Spread and Affected Species

CCHFV has a broad reach concerning its transmission and host range. Typically, transmission to humans occurs through the bite of an infected tick or direct contact with contaminated animal fluids [9]. The virus has a versatile host range, infecting animals such as livestock and small mammals, usually without causing apparent illness. In stark contrast, CCHFV can cause a grievous hemorrhagic fever in humans, with mortality rates that can soar as high as 30%, affecting populations across more than 30 countries [20].

Genetic Complexity and Evolution

The Crimean-Congo hemorrhagic fever virus stands out for its remarkable genetic diversity among tick-borne viruses. It is not uncommon for various strains to exhibit distinct nucleotide sequences, even within a defined location [20]. Interestingly, strains that closely resemble each other genetically have been found far apart across the globe. Ticks may facilitate the spread of the virus over long distances by hitching rides on migratory birds or through the movement of livestock in international trade [21]. Additionally, when coinfection occurs – where ticks or animals are infected with multiple strains of the virus simultaneously – it is thought that genetic mixing, or 'reassortment', can occur. This process might contribute to the vast diversity observed in the virus's genetic makeup [22].

Certain tick species primarily carry and spread the Crimean-Congo hemorrhagic fever virus, acting as carriers and reservoirs for the virus, usually without showing any symptoms themselves. The primary ticks responsible are:

1. *Hyalomma lusitanicum:* This species is critical for spreading the CCHFV and plays an essential role in keeping the virus circulating in the environment [23].
2. *Hyalomma marginatum:* This tick is notably involved in the virus's lifecycle,

especially within the Western Palearctic zone, which includes countries like Turkey [16, 23].

3. ***Hyalomma aegyptium:*** This tick is also known to harbor the virus while looking for a host to feed on and while feeding. Additionally, this tick can carry the virus in tortoises, suggesting there might be hidden or less obvious ways the virus spreads [24].

These tick species help keep the virus going by facilitating 'silent' transmission cycles between the ticks and their animal hosts.

CCHF: The Disease and its Transmission Cycle

The Crimean-Congo Hemorrhagic Fever Virus [CCHFV] is a tick-borne virus from the Nairoviridae family within the Bunyavirales order. An enveloped, negative-sense RNA virus belongs to the Orthonairovirus genus. CCHFV is part of the Bunyaviridae family, which includes over 350 identified isolates across five genera: Hantavirus, Nairovirus, Orthobunyavirus, Phlebovirus, and Tospovirus [9].

The genome of CCHFV comprises three RNA segments: Small [S], Medium [M], and Large [L]. The S segment codes for the Nucleocapsid Protein [N], the M segment codes for the viral glycoproteins, and the L segment codes for an RNA-dependent RNA polymerase [RdRp; the L protein], providing essential information about the viral genome's functional components [18, 25]. Each segment fulfills a specific coding function within the virus. These segments encode the viral proteins, and compared to other viruses within the order that causes human disease, CCHFV has a more intricate genomic structure. Classifying CCHFV as a biosafety level 3 or 4 pathogen varies by country, making clinical diagnosis potentially dangerous. The virus is geographically widespread due to the extensive range of its tick vectors, which are present in approximately 30 countries across Africa, Asia, the Middle East, and southern Europe [1, 20].

The primary transmission route for Crimean-Congo Hemorrhagic Fever [CCHF] is through tick bites, especially from ticks belonging to the "*Hyalomma*" genus. These ticks are vital in transmitting the CCHF Virus [CCHFV] among ticks and mammals, as well as through co-feeding among ticks. Species within the "*Hyalomma*" genus are notable vectors for various pathogens, including CCHFV, making them significant in disease transmission [24, 26].

Climate change is anticipated to increasingly favor the thriving of xerophilous *Hyalomma* ticks in dry conditions, potentially increasing their prevalence and disease transmission risk. These ticks are crucial in spreading diseases like CCHF between animals and humans, emphasizing their significance in the epidemiology of tick-borne illnesses [27].

In summary, tick bites from the "*Hyalomma*" genus are the main transmission route for CCHF, highlighting these ticks' essential role in spreading the disease between animals and humans.

Hyalomma genus

The primary transmission route for Crimean-Congo Hemorrhagic Fever [CCHF] is through tick bites from the "*Hyalomma*" genus, which are the main vectors of the CCHF virus [14]. Ticks and mammals sustain this virus through a two-year transmission cycle, involving both vertical and horizontal transmission among ticks and mammals, as well as direct transmission between ticks during co-feeding [17, 24].

Hyalomma genus ticks serve as reservoirs and vectors for the CCHF virus. The larvae and nymphs of *Hyalomma* ticks typically feed on hares and small birds, while adult ticks feed on larger animals such as cattle, sheep, and other large animals [5]. The pathogen is transmitted to humans through bites from infected ticks and contact with infected animals. It can also spread between humans in hospital settings, known as nosocomial transmission [24]. Human-to-human transmission can also occur through exposure to infectious bodily fluids from an infected individual or through contact with blood or products derived from infected animals. Migrating birds can transport infected ticks, aiding in the dispersal of the virus [23, 28]. The tick's life cycle and the virus transmission pathway involve the larvae feeding on small animals, molting into nymphs and adults, feeding on larger animals, and mating while attached to their host [29].

Vertical transmission happens when the virus replicates within the tick's tissues during metamorphosis and is passed on to the eggs and adult ticks from infected adult females and males, respectively. This transovarial transmission produces thousands of infected eggs, maintaining a large population of infected ticks [19, 29].

In summary, the primary transmission route for CCHF is through bites from infected *Hyalomma* ticks. The virus maintains itself *via* a complex cycle involving ticks and mammals, with co-feeding and contact with infected animals and humans facilitating vertical and horizontal transmission.

Replication Cycle of CCHFV

Entry: The virus infiltrates host cells *via* receptor-mediated endocytosis, liberating itself from the endosome to access the cytoplasm [2].

Transcription: The viral RNA-dependent RNA polymerase [RdRp] transcribes the negative-sense RNA genome into positive-sense RNA [30].

Positive-sense RNA transforms into viral proteins, including the Nucleocapsid Protein [NP], glycoproteins [Gn and Gc], and RNA-dependent RNA polymerase [RdRp] [12].

Replication: The virus replicates its genome using viral proteins, synthesizing new viral RNA, and assembling new viral particles [12, 25].

Assembly: Newly formed viral particles are constructed and released from the host cell, a process facilitated by viral glycoproteins [Gn and Gc] [31].

The Interaction Between Cchfv and Host Cells is Pivotal for Viral Replication and Pathogenesis

Apoptosis: The virus triggers apoptosis in host cells, potentially aiding viral replication and dissemination [32].

Host Cell Signaling: CCHFV influences host cell signaling pathways, impacting the host immune response and disease progression [33].

Host Cell Proteins: The virus interacts with host cell proteins, such as nucleolin, contributing to viral entry and replication [34].

Transmission Routes

Transmission routes for Crimean-Congo Hemorrhagic Fever [CCHF] encompass contact with contaminated blood or bodily fluids, and although uncommon, inhalation is also a potential route [35]. Human infection can occur through direct exposure to the blood or bodily fluids of infected individuals. Documented cases of nosocomial transmission in hospitals have occurred due to improper sterilization of medical equipment, reuse of injection needles, and contamination of medical supplies [36]. Although the main transmission route involves contact with infected ticks or animal blood, the possibility of human-to-human transmission *via* exposure to infectious body fluids highlights the need for stringent infection control protocols [37]. These measures are essential for preventing the dissemination of CCHF within healthcare environments and among individuals in close contact with infected persons [14].

The clinical presentation of Crimean-Congo Hemorrhagic Fever [CCHF] varies from mild flu-like symptoms to severe, life-threatening complications, typically progressing through four stages: incubation, pre-hemorrhagic, hemorrhagic, and healing.

Incubation Period

Symptoms begin suddenly 1-3 days after a tick bite or 5-6 days after exposure to infected blood or tissues [38].

Pre-Hemorrhagic Stage

Symptoms encompass fever, muscle discomfort, vertigo, neck and back pain, headaches, eye soreness, and sensitivity to light [photophobia]. Gastrointestinal issues, such as nausea, vomiting, diarrhea, and abdominal discomfort, are prevalent, often accompanied by a sore throat [39]. Patients may also experience mood changes, disorientation, drowsiness, and feelings of melancholy. Other signs include upper right quadrant abdominal pain, an enlarged liver [hepatomegaly], rapid heart rate [tachycardia], and enlarged lymph nodes [lymphadenopathy]. A petechial rash may appear on mucosal surfaces and the skin [34, 35].

Hemorrhagic Stage

Petechiae can progress to more extensive rashes, known as ecchymoses, and other bleeding phenomena. Signs of hepatitis may be present. Rapid deterioration of kidney function, sudden liver failure, or pulmonary failure may occur after the fifth day of illness. Patients continue to experience fever, headache, generalized body pain, nausea, vomiting, diarrhea, and tachycardia [26, 39].

Complications

Severe complications include extensive bleeding and bruising [ecchymoses]. Hemorrhagic symptoms, more frequent in fatal cases, include nosebleeds [epistaxis], gastrointestinal bleeding, bloody diarrhea, widespread bruising, rash, gum bleeding, petechiae, ecchymosis, and blood in the urine [hematuria]. Longer Prothrombin Time [PT] is significantly associated with fatal outcomes [40, 41].

In summary, CCHF initially presents with sudden fever, headache, muscle pain, weakness, fatigue, dizziness, neck pain, backache, sore eyes, photophobia, and nausea. As the disease progresses, patients may develop a petechial rash, ecchymoses, and hemorrhagic complications that can lead to organ failure and death in severe cases. Supportive care and early treatment with ribavirin are crucial for managing the disease.

Specific Treatment and the Importance of Supportive Care

While there is no definitive treatment for Crimean-Congo Hemorrhagic Fever [CCHF], supportive care is essential for managing the disease and reducing mortality. The antiviral ribavirin may be beneficial, particularly when administered early in the illness, but its effectiveness remains debated [42]. Without a cure, treatment focuses on supportive care, which includes maintaining fluid and electrolyte balance, monitoring and correcting coagulation issues, and managing complications such as bleeding and secondary infections. Patients with severe complications may need intensive care, including ventilatory support [1, 2]. The absence of well-equipped intensive care units in some healthcare settings contributes to higher mortality rates among CCHF patients. Therefore, timely hospital admission and prompt initiation of supportive treatments are critical for improving outcomes [43].

In summary, although specific treatments for CCHF are limited, providing thorough supportive care tailored to each patient's needs is crucial for managing the disease and reducing the risk of complications and death. Enhancing healthcare infrastructure and incredibly intensive care capabilities can improve survival rates among CCHF patients.

Link Between Rising Temperatures and Tick Populations [Development, Survival, Reproduction].

The relationship between rising temperatures and tick populations is complex and multifaceted. While the effects of climate change on argasid tick development are not well understood, temperature and humidity significantly influence the timing and rate of egg laying [oviposition], egg viability, and female tick longevity [44]. Studies have shown that temperature affects other tick species' development, survival, reproduction [fecundity], and behavior. Higher temperatures can accelerate the development and replication rates of tick-borne pathogens, potentially increasing the risk of transmission. Research on Theileria parva, which causes East Coast fever in cattle, suggests that elevated temperatures can shorten the transmission processing time for the pathogen in infected ticks [45].

Similarly, higher average temperatures during the summer and autumn can increase the virus load in infected *I. ricinus* ticks, raising the relative risk of human disease following an infected tick bite during warmer weather [46]. Temperature also impacts tick egg productivity and hatch rates. The number of eggs laid per mg of body weight decreases significantly at lower temperatures, and hatch rates drop as temperatures decline. Critical low temperatures for oviposition, egg hatching, and molting of larvae and nymphs have been identified for particular tick species, indicating that temperatures below these thresholds can severely affect tick development and survival [27, 44].

Additionally, climate-driven changes in host populations can lead to increased tick abundance. For example, warmer conditions can increase food availability for rodents, which serve as hosts for immature ticks, resulting in higher tick populations. Changes in human behavior, such as increased outdoor activities in warmer weather, also contribute to higher incidences of tick-borne infections [24, 44].

In summary, rising temperatures can influence tick populations by accelerating the development and replication of tick-borne pathogens, increasing tick abundance through changes in host populations, and altering tick behavior to avoid desiccation. These factors collectively raise the risk of tick-borne diseases in humans.

Altered Precipitation Patterns of Ticks

Altered precipitation patterns due to climate change can significantly expand the suitable habitats for ticks that transmit Crimean-Congo Hemorrhagic Fever [CCHF]. Here is how these changes can contribute to the expansion of tick habitats for CCHF transmission:

1. **Increased Moisture and Humidity:** Changes in precipitation can lead to higher moisture and humidity levels in certain regions, creating more favorable conditions for tick survival and reproduction. Ticks thrive in humid environments, and increased precipitation provides the necessary moisture for ticks to complete their life cycle [23, 47].
2. **Extended Questing Periods:** Altered precipitation patterns can affect the questing behavior of ticks, which involves climbing vegetation to wait for a host. With more moisture from increased precipitation, ticks can remain hydrated longer, extending their questing periods and increasing the chances of encountering and attaching to hosts [48].
3. **Expanded Geographic Range:** Changes in precipitation can alter the geographic range of ticks carrying the CCHF virus. Regions previously unsuitable for tick habitation due to low moisture levels may become suitable with increased precipitation. This expansion can lead to the migration of tick populations to new areas, raising the risk of CCHF transmission in previously unaffected regions [46, 48].
4. **Host Availability:** Precipitation changes can impact the availability of hosts for ticks. Altered precipitation influences vegetation growth, which in turn affects the abundance of host animals, such as rodents and livestock. An

increase in host populations due to changes in vegetation can provide more opportunities for ticks to feed and reproduce, leading to higher tick numbers and potentially spreading CCHF [44, 49].

In conclusion, altered precipitation patterns from climate change can create more conducive environments for ticks that transmit CCHF by increasing moisture levels, extending questing periods, expanding their geographic range, and enhancing host availability. These changes can lead to increased tick populations and the potential spread of CCHF to new areas previously unaffected by tick infestations.

Migratory Birds Disperse Infected Ticks to new Regions

Migratory birds significantly contribute to the spread of infected *"Hyalomma"* ticks to new regions, especially in climate-induced changes in migration patterns. These birds travel long distances during their seasonal migrations, potentially introducing tick and pathogen species into areas where they previously did not exist [50]. Climate and environmental changes can alter bird behaviors, subsequently affecting the distribution and prevalence of ticks and tick-borne pathogens [50, 51].

Research indicates that migratory birds can carry various tick species, including those from the *Hyalomma marginatum* group, known to transmit Crimean-Congo Hemorrhagic Fever [CCHF]. Bird species that spend more time on the ground in search of food have higher tick infestation rates, closely linking the geographic distribution of these ticks to their migratory routes [17]. Due to their ground-dwelling behavior and high tick infestation rates, species like the Whinchat and Common Whitethroat are particularly significant in introducing ticks into new areas.

The dispersal of ticks and tick-borne pathogens by migratory birds has essential ecological, medical, and veterinary implications. As the climate changes, tick distribution and abundance may increase in certain regions, potentially leading to the establishment of new tick populations and the spread of tick-borne diseases. The introduction of pathogens and vector species, the abundance of vectors and hosts, and the adaptation of pathogens to new vectors and vertebrate hosts are critical factors in the dispersal and establishment of vector-borne infections [17, 52].

In summary, migratory birds play a crucial role in spreading infected *Hyalomma* ticks to new areas, and climate-induced changes in migration patterns can facilitate this process. Understanding the complex mechanisms behind the emergence of vector-borne zoonoses, including the role of migratory birds, is essential for developing strategies to mitigate the risk of tick-borne diseases.

Potential Impact of Land-Use Changes on Tick-Human Contact

Land-use changes can significantly increase the risk of Crimean-Congo Hemorrhagic Fever [CCHF] by enhancing the contact between CCHF-causing ticks and humans. Key ways in which land-use changes influence this contact include:

1. **Deforestation and Habitat Fragmentation:** Converting core wildlife habitats into agricultural or urban areas creates more edge habitats. This transition leads to increased encounters between ticks, humans, and livestock as wildlife enters human-dominated areas in search of food or to traverse fragmented habitats [53].
2. **Urbanization:** Expanding urban areas into undeveloped land increases human proximity to tick habitats, raising the likelihood of tick bites and CCHF transmission. Researchers have observed this pattern as a factor contributing to the occurrence of CCHF in areas such as Gujarat, India [46, 54].
3. **Agricultural Expansion:** Turning natural habitats into croplands or pastures can change the composition of host species, often favoring those that support tick populations capable of transmitting CCHF. For example, higher densities of buffalo, a known livestock host, have been identified as a risk factor for CCHF in spatial risk assessments for Gujarat and India [13, 50].
4. **Altered Microclimate:** Land-use changes, such as increased humidity or suitable vegetation cover, can affect local microclimates to enhance tick survival and reproduction. Over the past 110 years, variations in maximum temperature have been linked to CCHF occurrences in affected districts of Gujarat [55].

In summary, changes in land use that create more edge habitats, bring humans closer to tick habitats, alter host species composition, or modify microclimates to benefit ticks can significantly increase the risk of CCHF by facilitating more excellent contact between ticks and humans.

The Connection Between Climate Change and Outbreaks of CCHF

Several research studies have highlighted the connection between climate change and epidemics of Crimean-Congo Hemorrhagic Fever [CCHF]:

1. **Gujarat, India Study:** Research in Gujarat identified that land use changes and increases in maximum temperature in affected districts were significant

contributors to CCHF occurrences. Spatial risk maps highlighted buffalo density, minimum land surface temperature, and elevation as key risk factors [56].

2. **Long-term Temperature Analysis in India:** A study examining temperature changes over 110 years in India found notable change points linked to CCHF outbreaks. The combination of land-use changes, increased temperatures, buffalo density, and elevation contributed to the emergence and spread of CCHF in this region [14, 56].

3. **Geographic Range of Ticks:** Research has demonstrated that climate change can expand the geographic range of ticks carrying the CCHF virus. Previously unsuitable areas may become viable habitats due to increased precipitation, leading to the migration of tick populations and an elevated risk of CCHF transmission [27].

4. **Role of Migratory Birds:** Migratory birds significantly contribute to the spread of infected *Hyalomma* ticks to new regions. Climate change can alter migration patterns, facilitating the establishment of new tick populations and further spreading CCHF [52].

5. **Impact of Land-use Changes:** Changes in land use that create more edge habitats, bring humans closer to tick habitats, alter host species composition, or modify microclimates favorable for ticks can significantly increase the risk of CCHF by enhancing contact between ticks and humans [17, 56].

In summary, various studies provide evidence linking climate change—through changes in temperature, precipitation patterns, and land use—to the emergence and spread of CCHF outbreaks in different regions. Addressing the public health challenges posed by CCHF necessitates a multifaceted approach that considers the complex interactions between climate change, environmental factors, and disease transmission dynamics.

Potential Burden of Increased CCHF Outbreaks Due to Climate Change

Climate change is expected to significantly increase the global burden of Crimean-Congo Hemorrhagic Fever (CCHF), a deadly viral disease transmitted by ticks and spreading to new areas, likely due to climatic shifts [51]. The prevalence of CCHF and other arboviral diseases is projected to rise with changing climate conditions. Factors facilitating the spread of CCHF include hot, humid climates, limited pesticide use, inadequate animal control, poor irrigation practices, and deficiencies in vector control. For instance, heavy monsoon seasons in Pakistan have been linked to a surge in CCHF cases due to improper irrigation, creating ideal environments for ticks [50, 51].

Researchers believe changes in the biology and geographical distribution of tick vectors in Sudan contribute to the emergence and spread of CCHF into new areas. CCHF outbreaks in Sudan have affected multiple states, with the largest outbreak in 2010 spanning five states [19]. Most cases occur between September and January, aligning with the rainy season when livestock are moved to open pastures, increasing tick abundance. Globally, researchers do not have a clear understanding of the burden of CCHF. Still, they recognize it as the most widespread tick-borne viral infection and a significant hemorrhagic fever disease [39]. In Africa, from 2003 to 2018, there were 62 reported CCHF cases with a 40% fatality rate. In Pakistan, the disease re-emerges annually, with six deaths reported by June 2023 in the latest wave [1].

To address the growing threat of CCHF due to climate change, experts recommend raising public awareness, improving irrigation practices, establishing surveillance systems, implementing livestock quarantine and vaccination, and investing in research for treatments and vaccines [42]. An integrated One Health approach, considering human, animal, and environmental health, is necessary to mitigate the threat of CCHF and other emerging infectious diseases driven by climate change [34, 53]. Public awareness and education are crucial in combating the growing threat of Crimean-Congo Hemorrhagic Fever [CCHF] outbreaks driven by climate change.

Importance of Public Awareness and Education about CCHF

Awareness of CCHF is the foundation of any health education effort. Understanding the causes, transmission methods, and preventive measures is crucial for increasing awareness and controlling the spread of the disease [57]. However, studies in Pakistan revealed that about half the population had never heard of "Congo fever." Among those who were aware, 79.8% had poor knowledge about the disease. The lack of education is a significant factor in the spread of CCHF. In Pakistan's Balochistan province, where most CCHF cases occur, the majority of people are illiterate and work as shepherds [30, 58]. They have insufficient knowledge, attitudes, and practices to prevent the disease. Even healthcare workers in Balochistan need a better understanding of CCHF due to a need for more skilled staff and resources. Preventive measures are scarce in Pakistan due to inadequate infrastructure, limited education, and restricted access to healthcare and livestock facilities [54, 57]. Experts recommend that Pakistan's health, agriculture, and media sectors collaborate with international organizations to create a strategic CCHF awareness and prevention framework.

Raising public awareness through education campaigns is crucial in combating CCHF. In Kazakhstan, officials plan to intensify prevention campaigns in regions affected by CCHF to educate people on how to minimize their risk when interacting with livestock. A Knowledge, Attitudes, and Practices [KAP] survey in Kazakhstan showed that combining this approach with serosurveys helped identify behaviors that increase CCHF transmission risk [57, 59].

In conclusion, enhancing public awareness about CCHF transmission, symptoms, and prevention is crucial to mitigating the growing burden of CCHF outbreaks exacerbated by climate change. Targeted education campaigns, particularly in high-risk areas, can empower communities to adopt safer practices and slow the spread of this deadly disease.

Crimean-Congo Hemorrhagic Fever [CCHF] is a severe viral disease that poses significant public health challenges due to its widespread geographic distribution, potential for rapid spread, and high mortality rate.

CCHF Diagnosis and its Available Treatments

Emphasizing the need for improved diagnostics and readily available treatments is crucial for several reasons:

Urgency of Improved Diagnostics

Early Detection and Containment: Early and accurate diagnosis is crucial for containing outbreaks, as CCHF can spread rapidly through human-to-human transmission, particularly in healthcare settings [60].

Symptom Overlap: The initial symptoms of CCHF are similar to many other febrile illnesses, making it difficult to distinguish without specific diagnostic tests [42].

Laboratory Safety: Current diagnostic methods often require sophisticated laboratory infrastructure and high biosafety precautions, highlighting the need for simpler, safer, and more accessible tests [61].

Need for Readily Available Treatments

High Mortality Rate: CCHF has a high case fatality rate, often ranging from 10% to 40%, emphasizing the need for effective treatments to reduce mortality [62].

Supportive Care Limitations: Supportive care is essential but limited, as patient outcomes largely depend on the body's ability to fight the virus [63].

Antiviral Research: Although limited antiviral drugs, such as ribavirin, have shown some efficacy, their availability and effectiveness vary, underscoring the need for further research and development [64].

Global Health Security

Preventing Epidemics: Improved diagnostics and treatments are essential for avoiding CCHF from spreading internationally and protecting populations worldwide [65].

Resource-Limited Settings: Ensuring that diagnostics and treatments are affordable and accessible in resource-limited settings is crucial to managing and controlling the disease [66].

Research and Development

Investment in R&D: Increased investment in research and development for CCHF diagnostics and treatments is necessary, including funding for the development of new technologies and the improvement of existing ones [28].

Collaborative Efforts: Collaborative efforts between governments, international health organizations, and the private sector can accelerate the development and distribution of diagnostics and treatments [44].

In summary, addressing the need for improved CCHF diagnostics and readily available treatments is a public health priority that requires concerted efforts to enhance diagnostic capabilities, develop effective treatments, and ensure accessibility in all affected regions. By doing so, we can better manage and control CCHF outbreaks, ultimately saving lives and improving global health security.

Strengthening surveillance systems for Crimean-Congo Hemorrhagic Fever [CCHF] in humans and animals is crucial for managing and controlling the disease. Effective surveillance can lead to early detection, timely response, and prevention of outbreaks, ultimately protecting public health. Here are vital points to advocate for enhanced surveillance systems:

Importance of Strengthened Surveillance Systems

Early Detection of Outbreaks: Enhanced surveillance systems enable the early detection of CCHF cases in humans and animals, facilitating prompt public health responses and reducing the spread of the virus [42].

Understanding Disease Epidemiology: Robust surveillance provides valuable data on the epidemiology of CCHF, including transmission patterns, geographic distribution, and seasonal trends, essential for developing targeted interventions and improving our understanding of the disease dynamics [42, 60].

Monitoring Animal Reservoirs: Surveillance in animal populations can identify areas where the virus is circulating, allowing for proactive measures to prevent spillover into human populations [58].

Critical Components of Effective Surveillance Systems

Integrated One Health Approach: Implementing a One Health approach that integrates human, animal, and environmental health is crucial for comprehensive surveillance, enhancing information sharing, and coordinated responses to CCHF [33, 34].

Enhanced Diagnostic Capabilities: Strengthening laboratory capacities to accurately and rapidly diagnose CCHF in humans and animals is essential, including training personnel, providing necessary equipment, and ensuring access to reliable diagnostic tests [28].

Data Collection and Reporting: Establishing standardized protocols for data collection, reporting, and analysis is vital for effective surveillance, facilitating timely interventions and resource allocation [65].

Tick Surveillance and Control: Monitoring tick populations and implementing control measures in high-risk areas can reduce the transmission of CCHF. These measures include tick density assessments, identification of tick species, and monitoring for the CCHF virus [66].

Benefits of Strengthened Surveillance

Improved Public Health Response: With robust surveillance, public health authorities can respond more effectively to CCHF cases and outbreaks, including implementing quarantine measures, providing targeted medical care, and conducting public awareness campaigns [26].

Prevention and Control: Surveillance data can inform the development of prevention and control strategies, such as vaccination programs for livestock, tick control measures, and public health education on reducing exposure risks [26, 37].

Resource Allocation: Accurate surveillance data enable efficient resource allocation, ensuring that areas with the highest risk of CCHF receive the necessary support for prevention, diagnosis, and treatment [67].

Global Health Security: Strengthened surveillance systems contribute to global health security by preventing the spread of CCHF across borders and facilitating international cooperation and data sharing for coordinated efforts to manage and control the disease globally [53, 68].

Advocacy Actions

Policy Development: Advocate for policies that support the establishment and maintenance of comprehensive CCHF surveillance systems, including funding for public health infrastructure, research, and capacity building [69].

Stakeholder Engagement: Engage stakeholders, including governments, international health organizations, and the private sector, to prioritize CCHF surveillance, leveraging resources and expertise to enhance surveillance capabilities [45].

Public Awareness: Raise awareness about the importance of CCHF surveillance among the general public and healthcare professionals, educating communities on recognizing symptoms and reporting cases to improve surveillance accuracy and timeliness [59].

Research and Innovation: Support research into new technologies and methods for CCHF surveillance, such as digital health tools, remote sensing, and predictive modeling, to enhance the efficiency and effectiveness of surveillance [43].

In conclusion, strengthening surveillance systems for CCHF in humans and animals is crucial for early detection, effective response, and prevention of outbreaks. By advocating for comprehensive surveillance approaches, we can protect public health, improve disease management, and enhance global health security.

Surveillance Systems for Crimean-Congo Hemorrhagic Fever [CCHF] in Humans and Animals

Several key strategies can be utilized to advocate for enhanced surveillance systems for Crimean-Congo Hemorrhagic Fever [CCHF] in humans and animals.

Standardized Case Definitions

Develop and apply standardized case definitions for reporting CCHF cases and tracing contacts in human and animal surveillance systems. This standardization enables consistent case reporting across different regions and facilitate the swift detection and confirmation of cases [3, 15].

Enhanced Laboratory Capacity

Build and maintain robust laboratory capacity in endemic areas and regions where the virus is likely to spread. Clinicians can support early treatment decisions by developing and utilizing rapid diagnostic tests [31, 60].

Vector Surveillance

Identify areas at risk for vector establishment by considering climatic and ecological conditions. Strengthen vector surveillance in these regions to predict human risk for CCHF and other tick-borne diseases [14].

Public Awareness and Education

Increase awareness of disease detection in rural areas, nosocomial transmission, and tick bite risks. Educate the public on safely and quickly removing ticks and using repellents appropriately [56].

Interdisciplinary Collaboration

Promote collaboration between the animal and human health sectors, as well as with international partners such as the WHO and OIE. Develop a national network of local, state, public health, hospital-based, and veterinary laboratories to respond to public health emergencies and provide CCHF diagnostics [66].

Digital Surveillance Systems

Implement digital surveillance systems that transmit information about zoonotic disease occurrences or suspicions from communities, such as *via* mobile phones or other digital platforms. These efforts can aid in early warning, diagnosis, and timely treatment of human cases at health centers [63].

Capacity Building and Training

Offer continuous training for healthcare workers on infection control precautions and recognizing high-risk procedures, especially in areas with high disease transmission risk [54].

Research and Development

Support vaccine development and further research on the curative use of ribavirin to enhance prevention and control measures for CCHF [53].

Implementing these strategies enhances surveillance systems for CCHF in humans and animals, resulting in more effective prevention, detection, and response to outbreaks of this severe disease [16].

Effective control programs for *Hyalomma* Ticks

Integrated Pest Management [IPM]

Adopt an IPM approach that integrates chemical, biological, genetic, ecological, and animal population selection methods to manage *Hyalomma* ticks. These strategies involve tailoring approaches to the local environment and specific tick species [34].

Acaricide Use

Apply acaricides judiciously, as *Hyalomma* ticks are developing resistance to many chemical treatments. Rotate different classes of acaricides to prevent the buildup of resistance [29].

Biological Control

Investigate biological control methods, such as using entomopathogenic fungi like *Alternaria sp.*, *Aspergillus*, and *Penicillium* to manage *Hyalomma* ticks in cattle. Further research is necessary to develop effective fungal biocontrol agents [37].

Tick-Resistant Livestock

Select and breed tick-resistant livestock to reduce infestations and pathogen transmission. This can be achieved through careful selection of animal populations [54].

Habitat Management

Manage tick habitats by clearing vegetation, fencing off high-risk areas, and using tick-repellent plants to reduce tick populations. Adapt habitat management practices to the local ecology of *Hyalomma* ticks [60].

Vaccination

Develop vaccines targeting conserved tick molecules to provide broad protection against *Hyalomma* ticks and the pathogens they transmit. Although promising, more research is needed to create effective vaccines [11].

Public Awareness

Raise awareness among livestock owners, farmers, and the public about diseases transmitted by *Hyalomma* ticks and the importance of tick control. Educate them on tick removal, the use of repellents, and reporting tick infestations [65].

Surveillance and Monitoring

Enhance surveillance systems to monitor *Hyalomma* tick populations, pathogen prevalence, and the effectiveness of control measures [29]. This will help guide decision-making and adjust control strategies as needed. By combining these strategies and tailoring them to local conditions, effective and sustainable *Hyalomma* tick control programs can be developed to protect human and animal health [24]. For International collaboration to address this global health threat, Continued Research on CCHF Diagnostics, Treatment, and Vaccines. To effectively combat Crimean-Congo Hemorrhagic Fever [CCHF], ongoing research is crucial to improve diagnostics, treatment, and vaccines [42]. Enhanced diagnostics are essential for early detection and accurate virus identification, which is vital for controlling outbreaks. Clinicians can use rapid diagnostic tests developed to support early treatment decisions [66].

Treatment

Investing in the development of effective treatments, including antiviral therapies such as ribavirin, is crucial to improving patient outcomes. The curative use of ribavirin remains further elucidated, and continued research is necessary to optimize treatment strategies [43].

International Collaboration

Addressing the threat of CCHF requires robust international collaboration. Collaborative efforts among countries and international organizations like the World Health Organization [WHO] and the World Organisation for Animal Health [OIE] are essential for tackling this global health threat. These efforts involve shared research, resources, and strategies to enhance surveillance, improve diagnostics, develop effective treatments and vaccines, and implement comprehensive tick control programs. Working together is pivotal in mitigating the impact of CCHF and safeguarding global health [33, 34].

Mathematical Models of CCHF

Mathematical modeling plays a crucial role in understanding the transmission dynamics of Crimean-Congo Hemorrhagic Fever [CCHF]. Various models have been developed to simulate the interactions among the virus, ticks, and hosts [humans and animals].

Compartmental Models

Ordinary Differential Equations [ODEs]: A common approach to model CCHF is through compartmental models using nonlinear ordinary differential equations. These models categorize populations into compartments such as susceptible, infected, and recovered individuals. The dynamics of the disease are described by a system of equations that represent the rates of transition between these compartments [70].

Basic Reproduction Number [R_0R_0]: This parameter is critical for understanding disease spread. It indicates the average number of secondary infections caused by one infected individual in a fully susceptible population. Models often calculate R_0 to assess potential outbreak risks [71].

Equilibrium Points: Stability analysis performed to identify equilibrium points of the system, which helps in understanding long-term behavior under different conditions [72].

Fractional-Order Models

Recent studies have introduced fractional-order models that incorporate historical memory effects into the transmission dynamics. For instance, a model utilizing the Caputo fractional-order derivative has been proposed, which enables more accurate simulations of CCHF transmission by accounting for past states of the system.

Model Characteristics

Historical Memory: This approach captures the influence of previous population states on current dynamics, providing a more nuanced understanding of transmission patterns [73].

Numerical Simulations: The Euler method is often employed to approximate solutions for these fractional systems, enabling researchers to visualize disease progression over time [54].

Tick-Borne Dynamics: Models focusing on tick-borne transmission have been developed to analyze how tick populations interact with hosts and contribute to CCHF outbreaks. These models consider factors such as tick density, host immunity, and environmental conditions influencing tick survival and transmission efficiency [26, 74].

Current Research on CCHF

Research on Crimean-Congo hemorrhagic fever [CCHF] has gained momentum due to the disease's significant public health impact and high case fatality rates.

Vaccine Development

Recent efforts have focused on creating effective vaccines against CCHF. A notable advancement is developing a nonhuman primate study model by a team from the National Institute of Allergy and Infectious Diseases [NIAID] [11, 56]. This model utilizes rhesus macaques as an alternative to cynomolgus macaques, previously prioritized for COVID-19 research. The aim is to facilitate the development of a replicating RNA-based vaccine against CCHF, which could significantly reduce the disease's impact in endemic regions [61].

Diagnostic Tools and Surveillance

The lack of practical diagnostic tools has been a significant hurdle in managing CCHF outbreaks. Current research emphasizes the need for improved serodiagnostic testing for humans and animals [16]. Enhanced surveillance protocols are also crucial for effectively monitoring CCHF transmission. Recent studies have highlighted the importance of intergovernmental coordination and the establishment of regional reference laboratories in strengthening diagnostic capabilities and response strategies.

Epidemiological Studies

Epidemiological research has been pivotal in understanding the transmission dynamics of CCHF. A recent spatial analysis identified 54 outbreaks across 414 districts in nine sub-Saharan African countries from 1981 to 2022, revealing patterns that can inform targeted interventions [75]. Additionally, a study reported a fatal case of CCHF in Portugal, underscoring the disease's geographic spread and the need for vigilant surveillance even in non-endemic areas [62].

One Health Approach

This multidisciplinary strategy aims to enhance cross-sectoral surveillance, develop novel interventions, and foster public awareness about risk factors associated with CCHF transmission. The approach emphasizes collaboration among various stakeholders to address the complexities of zoonotic diseases [74].

Public Health Challenges

Despite advancements in understanding CCHF, significant public health challenges persist. Cultural barriers, ineffective tick control measures, and limited healthcare infrastructure hinder effective prevention and response efforts. Research underscores the need for comprehensive public education campaigns to raise awareness about CCHF risks and preventive measures among at-risk populations [76, 77].

CONCLUSION

Crimean-Congo Hemorrhagic Fever [CCHF] presents a serious global health challenge that requires a multifaceted and cooperative approach to curb its spread effectively. The virus, mainly spread through tick bites, poses a substantial risk to the health of both humans and animals, resulting in elevated mortality rates and notable economic impacts. To mitigate these risks, adopting a comprehensive strategy that incorporates enhanced surveillance, improved diagnostics, effective treatments, and vaccination is crucial [1, 11, 56].

Robust surveillance is crucial for the early detection and accurate identification of CCHF cases, enabling swift and targeted interventions to control outbreaks. Enhanced diagnostics support early treatment decisions and identify the virus and its genetic variations. The presence of effective treatment options, such as antiviral therapies, is pivotal in enhancing patient outcomes and lowering mortality rates [1, 39]. Vaccination remains a key strategy in preventing the spread of CCHF and protecting at-risk populations. Developing vaccines that target conserved tick molecules could offer broad protection against current and emerging tick-borne pathogens [48].

International collaboration is vital for addressing the global threat of CCHF, which necessitates the exchange of research findings, resources, and strategies among nations and international entities like the World Health Organization [WHO] and the World Organisation for Animal Health [OIE] [52]. We can enhance surveillance, improve diagnostics, develop effective treatments and vaccines, and implement comprehensive tick control programs by working together. Such collective efforts are crucial for mitigating the impact of CCHF and ensuring global health security [11].

In summary, CCHF is a significant global health threat that demands a comprehensive and collaborative approach to combat. By implementing enhanced surveillance, improving diagnostics, providing effective treatment, and promoting vaccination, while fostering international cooperation, we can reduce the risk of transmission, enhance patient outcomes, and protect individuals and communities from this deadly disease.

REFERENCE

[1]   Ahmed A, Ali Y, Salim B, Dietrich I, Zinsstag J. Epidemics of Crimean-Congo Hemorrhagic Fever (CCHF) in Sudan between 2010 and 2020. Microorganisms 2022; 10(5): 928.
[http://dx.doi.org/10.3390/microorganisms10050928] [PMID: 35630372]

[2]   Omoga DCA, Tchouassi DP, Venter M, *et al.* Transmission dynamics of Crimean–Congo Haemorrhagic Fever Virus (CCHFV): Evidence of circulation in humans, livestock, and rodents in diverse ecologies in Kenya. Viruses 2023; 15(9): 1891.
[http://dx.doi.org/10.3390/v15091891] [PMID: 37766297]

[3]   Al-Abri SS, Abaidani IA, Fazlalipour M, *et al.* Current status of Crimean-Congo haemorrhagic fever in the World Health Organization Eastern Mediterranean Region: issues, challenges, and future directions. Int J Infect Dis 2017; 58: 82-9.
[http://dx.doi.org/10.1016/j.ijid.2017.02.018] [PMID: 28259724]

[4]   Bhuyan PJ, Nath AJ. Record of tropical rat mite, *ornithonyssus bacoti* (acari: Mesostigmata: Macronyssidae) from domestic and peridomestic rodents (*rattus rattus*) in nilgiris, Tamil Nadu, India. J Arthropod Borne Dis 2015; 10(1): 98-101.
[PMID: 27047977]

[5]   Bernard C, Holzmuller P, Bah MT, *et al.* Systematic review on crimean–congo hemorrhagic fever enzootic cycle and factors favoring virus transmission: Special focus on France, an apparently free-disease area in Europe. Front Vet Sci 2022; 9: 932304.
[http://dx.doi.org/10.3389/fvets.2022.932304] [PMID: 35928117]

[6]   Kuehnert PA, Stefan CP, Badger CV, Ricks KM. Crimean-Congo Hemorrhagic Fever Virus (CCHFV): A silent but widespread threat. Curr Trop Med Rep 2021; 8(2): 141-7.
[http://dx.doi.org/10.1007/s40475-021-00235-4] [PMID: 33747715]

[7]   Patel AA, Dalal YD, Parikh A, Gandhi R, Shah A. Crimean-Congo hemorrhagic fever: An emerging viral infection in India, revisited and lessons learned. Cureus 2023; 15(8): e43315.
[http://dx.doi.org/10.7759/cureus.43315] [PMID: 37700947]

[8]   Ergönül Ö. Crimean-Congo haemorrhagic fever. Lancet Infect Dis 2006; 6(4): 203-14.
[http://dx.doi.org/10.1016/S1473-3099(06)70435-2] [PMID: 16554245]

[9]   Shahhosseini N, Wong G, Babuadze G, *et al.* Crimean-congo hemorrhagic fever virus in Asia, Africa and Europe. Microorganisms 2021; 9(9): 1907.
[http://dx.doi.org/10.3390/microorganisms9091907] [PMID: 34576803]

[10]   Frank MG, Weaver G, Raabe V. Crimean-congo hemorrhagic fever virus for clinicians—diagnosis, clinical management, and therapeutics. Emerg Infect Dis 2024; 30(5): 864-73.
[http://dx.doi.org/10.3201/eid3005.231648] [PMID: 38666553]

[11]   Dowall SD, Carroll MW, Hewson R. Development of vaccines against Crimean-Congo haemorrhagic fever virus. Vaccine 2017; 35(44): 6015-23.
[http://dx.doi.org/10.1016/j.vaccine.2017.05.031] [PMID: 28687403]

[12]   Ma J, Guo Y, Gao J, *et al.* Climate change drives the transmission and spread of vector-borne diseases: An ecological perspective. Biology (Basel) 2022; 11(11): 1628.
[http://dx.doi.org/10.3390/biology11111628] [PMID: 36358329]

[13]   Vescio FM, Busani L, Mughini-Gras L, *et al.* Environmental correlates of crimean-congo haemorrhagic fever incidence in Bulgaria. BMC Public Health 2012; 12(1): 1116.
[http://dx.doi.org/10.1186/1471-2458-12-1116] [PMID: 23270399]

[14]   Fanelli A, Buonavoglia D. Risk of Crimean Congo Haemorrhagic Fever Virus (CCHFV) introduction

and spread in CCHF-free countries in southern and Western Europe: A semi-quantitative risk assessment. One Health 2021; 13: 100290.
[http://dx.doi.org/10.1016/j.onehlt.2021.100290] [PMID: 34307823]

[15]   Spengler JR, Bergeron É, Spiropoulou CF. Crimean-Congo hemorrhagic fever and expansion from endemic regions. Curr Opin Virol 2019; 34: 70-8.
[http://dx.doi.org/10.1016/j.coviro.2018.12.002] [PMID: 30660091]

[16]   Tahir I, Motwani J, Moiz MA, *et al.* Crimean-Congo hemorrhagic fever outbreak affecting healthcare workers in Pakistan: an urgent rising concern. Ann Med Surg (Lond) 2024; 86(6): 3201-3.
[http://dx.doi.org/10.1097/MS9.0000000000002127] [PMID: 38846901]

[17]   Santibáñez P, Palomar AM, Portillo A, Santibáñez S, Oteo JA, Santibáñez P, *et al.* The role of chiggers as human pathogens. An Overview of Tropical Diseases 2015. Available from: https://www.intechopen.com/chapters/49626
[http://dx.doi.org/10.5772/61978]

[18]   Bachmann PA, Gibbs EPJ, Murphy FA, Studdert MJ, White DO Structure and composition of viruses. Vet Virol 1987; pp. 3-19.

[19]   Kasson P, DiMaio F, Yu X, *et al.* Model for a novel membrane envelope in a filamentous hyperthermophilic virus. eLife 2017; 6: e26268.
[http://dx.doi.org/10.7554/eLife.26268] [PMID: 28639939]

[20]   Hawman DW, Feldmann H. Crimean–Congo haemorrhagic fever virus. Nat Rev Microbiol 2023; 21(7): 463-77.
[http://dx.doi.org/10.1038/s41579-023-00871-9] [PMID: 36918725]

[21]   Dobelmann J, Felden A, Lester PJ. Genetic strain diversity of multi-host RNA viruses that infect a wide range of pollinators and associates is shaped by geographic origins. Viruses 2020; 12(3): 358.
[http://dx.doi.org/10.3390/v12030358] [PMID: 32213950]

[22]   Fleischmann WR. Baron S, editor Medical Microbiology [Internet] 4th ed 1996. Available from: http://www.ncbi.nlm.nih.gov/books/NBK8439/

[23]   Keikha M. The discrepancy of Crimean-Congo hemorrhagic fever-related tick vectors: An urgent need for boosted surveillance. Ann Med Surg (Lond) 2022; 81: 104412.
[http://dx.doi.org/10.1016/j.amsu.2022.104412] [PMID: 36035598]

[24]   Kar S, Rodriguez SE, Akyildiz G, *et al.* Crimean-Congo hemorrhagic fever virus in tortoises and *Hyalomma aegyptium* ticks in East Thrace, Turkey: potential of a cryptic transmission cycle. Parasit Vectors 2020; 13(1): 201.
[http://dx.doi.org/10.1186/s13071-020-04074-6] [PMID: 32307010]

[25]   Carter SD, Surtees R, Walter CT, *et al.* Structure, function, and evolution of the Crimean-Congo hemorrhagic fever virus nucleocapsid protein. J Virol 2012; 86(20): 10914-23.
[http://dx.doi.org/10.1128/JVI.01555-12] [PMID: 22875964]

[26]   Sorvillo TE, Rodriguez SE, Hudson P, *et al.* Towards a sustainable one health approach to crimean–congo hemorrhagic fever prevention: Focus areas and gaps in knowledge. Trop Med Infect Dis 2020; 5(3): 113.
[http://dx.doi.org/10.3390/tropicalmed5030113] [PMID: 32645889]

[27]   Yılmaz S, İba Yilmaz S, Alay H, Koşan Z, Eren Z. Temporal tendency, seasonality and relationship with climatic factors of Crimean-Congo Hemorrhagic Fever cases (East of Turkey: 2012–2021). Heliyon 2023; 9(9): e19593.
[http://dx.doi.org/10.1016/j.heliyon.2023.e19593] [PMID: 37681169]

[28]   Biggs HM, Behravesh CB, Bradley KK, *et al.* Diagnosis and management of tickborne rickettsial diseases: Rocky mountain spotted fever and other spotted fever group rickettsioses, ehrlichioses, and anaplasmosis — United States. MMWR Recomm Rep 2016; 65(2): 1-44.
[http://dx.doi.org/10.15585/mmwr.rr6502a1] [PMID: 27172113]

[29] Knight MM, Norval RAI, Rechav Y. The life cycle of the tick Hyalomma marginatum rufipes Koch (Acarina: Ixodidae) under laboratory conditions. J Parasitol 1978; 64(1): 143-6.
[http://dx.doi.org/10.2307/3279627] [PMID: 627955]

[30] Boulant S, Stanifer M, Lozach PY. Dynamics of virus-receptor interactions in virus binding, signaling, and endocytosis. Viruses 2015; 7(6): 2794-815.
[http://dx.doi.org/10.3390/v7062747] [PMID: 26043381]

[31] Fair JM, Al-Hmoud N, Alrwashdeh M, *et al.* Transboundary determinants of avian zoonotic infectious diseases: challenges for strengthening research capacity and connecting surveillance networks. Front Microbiol 2024; 15: 1341842.
[http://dx.doi.org/10.3389/fmicb.2024.1341842] [PMID: 38435695]

[32] Obiegala A, Arnold L, Pfeffer M, *et al.* Host–parasite interactions of rodent hosts and ectoparasite communities from different habitats in Germany. Parasit Vectors 2021; 14(1): 112.
[http://dx.doi.org/10.1186/s13071-021-04615-7] [PMID: 33596984]

[33] Dai S, Min YQ, Li Q, *et al.* Interactome profiling of Crimean-Congo hemorrhagic fever virus glycoproteins. Nat Commun 2023; 14(1): 7365.
[http://dx.doi.org/10.1038/s41467-023-43206-1] [PMID: 37963884]

[34] Kumar D, Broor S, Rajala MS. Interaction of host nucleolin with influenza A virus nucleoprotein in the early phase of infection limits the late viral gene expression. PLoS One 2016; 11(10): e0164146.
[http://dx.doi.org/10.1371/journal.pone.0164146] [PMID: 27711134]

[35] Yagci-Caglayik D, Kayaaslan B, Yapar D, *et al.* Monitoring Crimean-Congo haemorrhagic fever virus RNA shedding in body secretions and serological status in hospitalised patients, Turkey, 2015. Euro Surveill 2020; 25(10): 1900284.
[http://dx.doi.org/10.2807/1560-7917.ES.2020.25.10.1900284] [PMID: 32183931]

[36] Monegro AF, Muppidi V, Regunath H. Hospital-Acquired Infections In: StatPearls 2024. Available from: http://www.ncbi.nlm.nih.gov/books/NBK441857/

[37] van Seventer JM, Hochberg NS. Principles of infectious diseases: Transmission, diagnosis, prevention, and control. Int Encycl Public Health 2017; pp. 22-39.
[http://dx.doi.org/doi: 10.1016/B978-0-12-803678-5.00516-6]

[38] Sadeghi M, Asgharzadeh SA, Bayani M, Alijanpour E, Javaniyan M, Jabbari A. Crimean congo hemorrhagic fever appearance in the north of Iran. Caspian J Intern Med 2013; 4(1): 617-20.
[PMID: 24009947]

[39] Salih N, Baig KS, Jan MA, *et al.* Crimean-congo hemorrhagic fever presented in dengue epidemic: A case report. Cureus 2023; 15(5): e39015.
[http://dx.doi.org/10.7759/cureus.39015] [PMID: 37323327]

[40] Gilmour MI. Increased Immune and Inflammatory Responses to Dust Mite Antigen in Rats Exposed to 5 ppm NO2

[41] Pietras NM, Pearson-Shaver AL. Immune Thrombocytopenic Purpura In: StatPearls 2024. Available from: http://www.ncbi.nlm.nih.gov/books/NBK562282/

[42] Papa A, Mirazimi A, Köksal I, Estrada-Pena A, Feldmann H. Recent advances in research on Crimean-Congo hemorrhagic fever. J Clin Virol 2015; 64: 137-43.
[http://dx.doi.org/10.1016/j.jcv.2014.08.029] [PMID: 25453328]

[43] Fabara SP, Ortiz JF, Smith DW, *et al.* Crimean-congo hemorrhagic fever beyond ribavirin: A systematic review. Cureus 2021; 13(9): e17842.
[PMID: 34557373]

[44] Gray JS, Dautel H, Estrada-Peña A, Kahl O, Lindgren E. Effects of climate change on ticks and tick-borne diseases in europe. Interdiscip Perspect Infect Dis 2009; 2009: 1-12.
[http://dx.doi.org/10.1155/2009/593232] [PMID: 19277106]

[45]   Fry LM, Schneider DA, Frevert CW, Nelson DD, Morrison WI, Knowles DP. East coast fever caused by theileria parva is characterized by macrophage activation associated with vasculitis and respiratory failure. PLoS One 2016; 11(5): e0156004.
        [http://dx.doi.org/10.1371/journal.pone.0156004] [PMID: 27195791]

[46]   Daniel M, Danielová V, Fialová A, Malý M, Kříž B, Nuttall PA. Increased relative risk of tick-borne encephalitis in warmer weather. Front Cell Infect Microbiol 2018; 8: 90.
        [http://dx.doi.org/10.3389/fcimb.2018.00090] [PMID: 29623261]

[47]   Beard CB, Eisen RJ, Barker CM, Garofalo JF, Hahn M, Hayden M, *et al.* Ch. 5: vectorborne diseases. The impacts of climate change on human health in the United States: a scientific assessment 2016; 129 56. Available from: https://health2016.globalchange.gov/vectorborne-diseases

[48]   Nielebeck C, Kim SH, Pepe A, *et al.* Climatic stress decreases tick survival but increases rate of host-seeking behavior. Ecosphere 2023; 14(1): e4369.
        [http://dx.doi.org/10.1002/ecs2.4369]

[49]   Davey RB. Effect of temperature on the ovipositional biology and egg viability of the cattle tickBoophilus annulatus (Acari: Ixodidae). Exp Appl Acarol 1988; 5(1-2): 1-14.
        [http://dx.doi.org/10.1007/BF02053812] [PMID: 3197576]

[50]   Buczek AM, Buczek W, Buczek A, Bartosik K. The potential role of migratory birds in the rapid spread of ticks and tick-borne pathogens in the changing climatic and environmental conditions in Europe. Int J Environ Res Public Health 2020; 17(6): 2117.
        [http://dx.doi.org/10.3390/ijerph17062117] [PMID: 32209990]

[51]   Nuttall PA. Climate change impacts on ticks and tick-borne infections. Biologia (Bratisl) 2022; 77(6): 1503-12. [Bratisl].
        [http://dx.doi.org/10.1007/s11756-021-00927-2]

[52]   Leblebicioglu H, Eroglu C, Erciyas-Yavuz K, Hokelek M, Acici M, Yilmaz H. Role of migratory birds in spreading Crimean-Congo hemorrhagic fever, Turkey. Emerg Infect Dis 2014; 20(8): 1331-4.
        [http://dx.doi.org/10.3201/eid2008.131547] [PMID: 25062428]

[53]   Wegner GI, Murray KA, Springmann M, *et al.* Averting wildlife-borne infectious disease epidemics requires a focus on socio-ecological drivers and a redesign of the global food system. EClinicalMedicine 2022; 47: 101386.
        [http://dx.doi.org/10.1016/j.eclinm.2022.101386] [PMID: 35465645]

[54]   Bhowmick S, Kasi KK, Gethmann J, *et al.* Ticks on the run: A mathematical model of crimean-congo haemorrhagic fever (CCHF)—key factors for transmission. Epidemiologia 2022; 3(1): 116-34.
        [http://dx.doi.org/10.3390/epidemiologia3010010] [PMID: 36417271]

[55]   Wimberly MC, Davis JK, Evans MV, *et al.* Land cover affects microclimate and temperature suitability for arbovirus transmission in an urban landscape. PLoS Negl Trop Dis 2020; 14(9): e0008614.
        [http://dx.doi.org/10.1371/journal.pntd.0008614] [PMID: 32956355]

[56]   Chanda MM, Kharkwal P, Dhuria M, *et al.* Quantifying the influence of climate, host and change in land-use patterns on occurrence of Crimean Congo Hemorrhagic Fever (CCHF) and development of spatial risk map for India. One Health 2023; 17: 100609.
        [http://dx.doi.org/10.1016/j.onehlt.2023.100609] [PMID: 37583365]

[57]   Jamil H, Din MFU, Tahir MJ, *et al.* Knowledge, attitudes, and practices regarding Crimean-Congo hemorrhagic fever among general people: A cross-sectional study in Pakistan. PLoS Negl Trop Dis 2022; 16(12): e0010988.
        [http://dx.doi.org/10.1371/journal.pntd.0010988] [PMID: 36480553]

[58]   Olson JG, Bourgeois AL, Fang RCY. Population indices of chiggers (Leptotrombidium deliense) and incidence of scrub typhus in Chinese military personnel, Pescadores Islands of Taiwan, 1976–1977. Trans R Soc Trop Med Hyg 1982; 76(1): 85-8.

[http://dx.doi.org/10.1016/0035-9203(82)90027-X] [PMID: 7080163]

[59] Ayebare D, Menya M, Mulyowa A, Muhwezi A, Tweyongyere R, Atim SA. Knowledge, attitudes, and practices of Crimean Congo hemorrhagic fever among livestock value chain actors in Kagadi district, Uganda. PLoS Negl Trop Dis 2023; 17(2): e0011107.
[http://dx.doi.org/10.1371/journal.pntd.0011107] [PMID: 36730376]

[60] Bartolini B, Gruber CEM, Koopmans M, *et al.* Laboratory management of Crimean-Congo haemorrhagic fever virus infections: perspectives from two European networks. Euro Surveill 2019; 24(5): 1800093.
[http://dx.doi.org/10.2807/1560-7917.ES.2019.24.5.1800093] [PMID: 30722811]

[61] Hawman DW, Feldmann H. Recent advances in understanding Crimean–Congo hemorrhagic fever virus. F1000Research. 2018 Oct 29;7:F1000. Fac Rev 1715.

[62] Belobo JTE, Kenmoe S, Kengne-Nde C, *et al.* Worldwide epidemiology of Crimean-Congo Hemorrhagic Fever Virus in humans, ticks and other animal species, a systematic review and meta-analysis. PLoS Negl Trop Dis 2021; 15(4): e0009299.
[http://dx.doi.org/10.1371/journal.pntd.0009299] [PMID: 33886556]

[63] Cascella M, Rajnik M, Aleem A, Dulebohn SC, Di Napoli R. Features, Evaluation, and Treatment of Coronavirus [COVID-19] In: StatPearls 2024. Available from: http://www.ncbi.nlm.nih.gov/books/NBK554776/

[64] Paintsil E, Cheng YC. Antiviral Agents. Encycl Microbiol 2009; pp. 223-57.

[65] Leblebicioglu H, Sunbul M, Memish ZA, *et al.* Consensus report: Preventive measures for Crimean-Congo Hemorrhagic Fever during Eid-al-Adha festival. Int J Infect Dis 2015; 38: 9-15.
[http://dx.doi.org/10.1016/j.ijid.2015.06.029] [PMID: 26183413]

[66] Land KJ, Boeras DI, Chen XS, Ramsay AR, Peeling RW. Reassured diagnostics to inform disease control strategies, strengthen health systems and improve patient outcomes. Nat Microbiol 2018; 4(1): 46-54.
[http://dx.doi.org/10.1038/s41564-018-0295-3] [PMID: 30546093]

[67] Messina JP, Pigott DM, Golding N, *et al.* The global distribution of Crimean-Congo hemorrhagic fever. Trans R Soc Trop Med Hyg 2015; 109(8): 503-13.
[http://dx.doi.org/10.1093/trstmh/trv050] [PMID: 26142451]

[68] Xu G, Walker DH, Jupiter D, Melby PC, Arcari CM. A review of the global epidemiology of scrub typhus. PLoS Negl Trop Dis 2017; 11(11): e0006062.
[http://dx.doi.org/10.1371/journal.pntd.0006062] [PMID: 29099844]

[69] McNabb SJN. Comprehensive effective and efficient global public health surveillance. BMC Public Health 2010; 10(Suppl 1) (Suppl. 1): S3.
[http://dx.doi.org/10.1186/1471-2458-10-S1-S3] [PMID: 21143825]

[70] Ramezani SB, Amirlatifi A, Rahimi S. A novel compartmental model to capture the nonlinear trend of COVID-19. Comput Biol Med 2021; 134: 104421.
[http://dx.doi.org/10.1016/j.compbiomed.2021.104421] [PMID: 33964736]

[71] Breban R, Vardavas R, Blower S. Theory versus data: how to calculate R0? PLoS One 2007; 2(3): e282.
[http://dx.doi.org/10.1371/journal.pone.0000282] [PMID: 17356693]

[72] Fornari C, Pin C, Yates JWT, Mettetal JT, Collins TA. Importance of stability analysis when using nonlinear semimechanistic models to describe drug-induced hematotoxicity. CPT Pharmacometrics Syst Pharmacol 2020; 9(9): 498-508.
[http://dx.doi.org/10.1002/psp4.12514] [PMID: 32453487]

[73] Skrip LA, Townsend JP. Modeling approaches toward understanding infectious disease transmission. Immunoepidemiology 2019; 227-43.
[http://dx.doi.org/10.1007/978-3-030-25553-4_14]

[74] Sorvillo TE, Rodriguez SE, Hudson P, *et al*. Towards a sustainable one health approach to crimean–congo hemorrhagic fever prevention: Focus areas and gaps in knowledge. Trop Med Infect Dis 2020; 5(3): 113.
[http://dx.doi.org/10.3390/tropicalmed5030113] [PMID: 32645889]

[75] Temur AI, Kuhn JH, Pecor DB, Apanaskevich DA, Keshtkar-Jahromi M. Epidemiology of crimean-congo hemorrhagic fever (CCHF) in Africa—underestimated for decades. Am J Trop Med Hyg 2021; 104(6): 1978-90.
[http://dx.doi.org/10.4269/ajtmh.20-1413] [PMID: 33900999]

[76] Okesanya OJ, Olatunji GD, Kokori E, *et al*. Looking beyond the lens of crimean-congo hemorrhagic fever in Africa. Emerg Infect Dis 2024; 30(7): 1319-25.
[http://dx.doi.org/10.3201/eid3007.230810] [PMID: 38916548]

[77] Asaaga FA, Young JC, Oommen MA, *et al*. Operationalising the "One Health" approach in India: facilitators of and barriers to effective cross-sector convergence for zoonoses prevention and control. BMC Public Health 2021; 21(1): 1517.
[http://dx.doi.org/10.1186/s12889-021-11545-7] [PMID: 34362321]

SUBJECT INDEX

A

Abdominal pain 98, 169
Abiotic elements 49, 58
Acaricides 72, 90, 181
Accidental hosts 25, 30, 36, 42, 71, 75
Aedes 2, 5, 7, 8, 94, 95, 96, 97, 100, 101,
    102, 103, 104, 105, 106, 107,
    108, 109, 110, 111, 113, 114,
    115, 117, 119, 128
   mosquitoes 2, 5, 7, 94, 96, 97, 101, 102,
    103, 104, 105, 106, 107, 108,
    109, 111, 113, 114, 115, 117,
    119, 128
   aegypti 8, 94, 95, 96, 97, 100, 101, 103,
    105, 106, 107, 108, 110
   albopictus 8, 94, 95, 97, 100, 101, 103,
    105, 106, 108, 109
Agent-based models 86, 116
Agricultural practices 3, 10, 40, 104, 145,
   150
Alkhurma hemorrhagic fever virus 69, 71
Anopheles 4, 14, 126, 127, 130, 132, 133,
    134, 135, 138, 141, 142, 143,
    147, 148, 151
   mosquitoes 4, 14, 126, 127, 130, 134,
    135, 138, 141, 142, 143, 147, 148
   arabiensis 141, 142, 143
   gambiae 141, 142, 143, 151
   stephensi 132, 133, 134
Anticoagulants 54, 136
Antimalarial drugs 132
Antimicrobial resistance 34
Antiviral medication 80, 163, 170
Arthropods 1, 21, 49
Asexual replication 137

B

Babesiosis 49
Basic reproduction number 42, 86, 115, 170

Behavior change communication 37
Biodiversity loss 60, 81
Biological control 12, 100, 181
Biphasic sickness 77
Biting behavior 3, 7, 105, 129
Blood meals 8, 54, 56, 100, 106, 135
Bonnet monkeys 69, 71, 76
Boophilus microplus 59, 67
Bunyavirales order 164, 166

C

Carbon sequestration 150
CCHF virus 162, 164, 166, 167, 168, 173
Chemical control 12
Chigger index 28
Chigger mites 10, 21-36
Chikungunya 2, 6, 14, 100, 110, 111, 112
Chills 6, 77
Co-feeding 166, 167
Co-infections 34, 110, 111, 112, 113
Compartmental models 183
Complications 10, 97, 138, 169
Culex mosquitoes 9, 27

D

Dead-end hosts 22, 71
Deforestation 2, 32, 48, 81, 104, 149
Dengue
   hemorrhagic fever 96, 97, 110, 111
   shock syndrome 96, 97, 110, 111
   virus 5, 7. 94, 95, 97, 103, 105, 106, 109,
    111, 114, 115, 116, 117
Diapause 48, 58
Diarrhea 69, 98, 169
Disease 1, 13, 14, 24, 48, 49, 59, 72, 97, 103,
    104, 105, 106, 107, 108, 109, 126, 129,
    147, 148, 154, 167
   surveillance 13, 49, 126, 148, 154

Jayalakshmi Krishnan, Sigamani Panneer, P. Thiyagarajan, Balachandar Vellingiri & Pradeep Kumar
Srivastava (Eds.)

www.ingramcontent.com/pod-product-compliance
Lightning Source LLC
Chambersburg PA
CBHW041658210326
41598CB00007B/456